Having completed a primary degree in psychology and a doctorate investigating the effects of drugs on behaviour, Arabella Melville rejected academic life. She turned instead to writing, and gained experience with the last rumblings of the Underground Press before going on to write articles for an assortment of magazines and newspapers. She collaborated with Colin Johnson in the writing of CURED TO DEATH and other books followed, taking them through a close examination of the nature of health.

She now divides her time between writing, gardening and assorted physical activities.

Colin Johnson has had a full and varied career. Developing interests in astronomy, cosmology, economics and history, he moved away from his work in industry. He has been involved in the field of constructional plastics, in the setting up of various co-operatives in Scotland and Wales, and has seen the rise and fall of his own business as a magazine and book distributor. Drawn into collaborating on CURED TO DEATH with partner Arabella, he now spends his time much as she does.

Hay Fever

Colin Johnson and
Arabella Melville

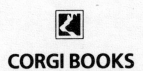

CORGI BOOKS

HAY FEVER

A CORGI BOOK 0 552 12480X 1

First publication in Great Britain

PRINTING HISTORY
Corgi edition published 1985

This book is set in

Corgi Books are published by
Transworld Publishers Ltd.,
Century House, 61–63 Uxbridge Road,
Ealing, London W5 5SA

Made and printed in Great Britain by the
Guernsey Press Co. Ltd., Guernsey, Channel Islands.

Acknowledgements

We should particularly like to thank Dr Michael Jenkins of the Royal London Homeopathic Hospital for the benefit of his time and expertise, and Dr David Reilly of Glasgow Homeopathic Hospital for generously offering to read our manuscript and making helpful suggestions.

We are grateful to Dr H.C. Masheter, Medical Director of Merrell Pharmaceuticals Limited, Mrs Josephine Saulter, Principal Medical Information Officer at Bencard, and Dr R.T. Owen, Advisory Pharmacologist at the Wellcome Foundation Limited, for supplying much useful background information. Dr John Mullins, of the Asthma Research Unit, Sully Hospital, S. Glamorgan, Felicity Jackson, of the Asthma and Allergy Treatment Research Centre, Derby, and Dr R. Davies, of St Mary's Hospital Medical School, Paddington, all responded to requests for information with great alacrity; their help proved invaluable. Thanks are also due to Mr Julian Laws of Medion Limited, Mr McCubbin of the Southeast Ionizer Centre, Dr Leslie Hawkins of Surrey University, and Martin Everett, an old personal friend, and an undoubted asset to the M.A.F.F.

And lastly, our heartfelt thanks to the homeopath in South Wales who first showed us that it is possible to live a life free from hay fever.

Contents

Introduction

The story of hay fever is one that spans thousands of years of human history. The disease seems to have had its origins in the stone age, at about the time humans settled to agriculture as a way of life.

Long before that other changes had forced plants to depend increasingly on the wind to carry pollen from one to another. To reproduce successfully in this random way enormous quantities of pollen had to be produced by each male flower.

These two changes set humans and plants on a collision course. With the addition of one more ingredient in the last few decades, the resulting crash has come to involve countless millions of people who now suffer from hay fever each spring and summer.

In exploring the precise nature of the disease we have to envisage the microscopic and molecular stage on which these events take place. It is in these minute interactions that they produce the sneezing and snuffling so dreaded by sufferers.

We found the exploration of the bodily processes involved both fascinating and amazing. We hope you capture some of our enthusiasm in the pursuit of an understanding of your particular hay fever problem.

While the condition may have some common major causes, when we consider each sufferer the disease rapidly becomes one of those ailments where every individual has their own particular version.

Hay fever is not an easy disease to get to grips with. If it was, no doubt a universal cure would have been found long ago. Understanding the cause, mechanism, and the possible courses of action that will alleviate it will demand more than simply finding something to stop the sneezing. Nevertheless, with a little patience and a wider understanding of the cause of the disease, that should be the end result of your efforts.

In discussing possible cures we have tried to be objective. We have no commercial interest to declare, we are writers with scientific backgrounds who specialise in books and articles concerned with health. We do not manufacture or market any of the products we discuss. The nearest we would get to bias may arise from the fact that one of us suffered from hay fever for almost thirty years before being treated by a homoeopath.

Doctors and specialists in a wide range of disciplines will all claim to the patient that their particular method is the only true science. That all others are little better than fakes or charlatans. These claims, from whatever source, have little to do with discovering what may be the best for each individual sufferer. We hope you will be sufficiently strong willed to ignore claims from the side-lines and concentrate on your own well-being.

Use this book to increase your understanding and wisdom, and to have faith in the judgement of your own needs. We believe it will act to guide you to your particular path to freedom from the misery of hay fever.

Colin Johnson, December 1983.

Hay Fever

1 Is it possible not to suffer at all?

For many people, the miseries of hay fever can be totally eliminated. And almost all hay fever sufferers can significantly reduce
the life-limiting effects of the disease.

This can only be good news for those who dread each summer,
the seemingly inevitable sneezes and swollen eyes, sore head and
running nose — symptoms that can feel worse than 'flu at the
hottest time of the year. Every year, millions of normally healthy
people rush to doctors and pharmacists for treatment in attempts
to alleviate these symptoms.

Although modern medicines can provide the answer for some,
most sufferers find them unsatisfactory. Either they fail to stop
the typical symptoms of hay fever, or they do so at an unacceptable cost in side-effects. Antihistamine tablets, the most widely
used type of remedy for hay fever, can put the sufferer to sleep —
which is clearly unacceptable when the aim in taking them was to
be able to lead a normal non-sneezing life. The drowsiness caused
by the effects of antihistamines on the brain is just one example
of a number of side-effects of hay fever treatments which limit
their usefulness.

What, then, is the answer? Unfortunately there isn't one simple remedy that will work for all hay fever sufferers. The cause
of the condition, the plant pollens that fill the air on those summer days when we want to be carefree in the sunshine, have many
sources. A wide variety of plants have been identified as causes of
the allergic response recognised as hay fever; and just as different
pollens will affect different people, so different ways of avoiding
suffering will be needed.

Another important contribution to the unique nature of the
disease for each sufferer is his or her own nature. The genes which
make us each different also produce an almost infinite number of

15

possible paths to allergic susceptibility. Both the individual factors and the number of pollens contribute to the difficulty of treating the condition.

Despite the variety of possible causes of hay fever, the effects on the cells of sufferers' bodies are much the same. The reactions vary in their degree of severity, depending on the quantity and type of pollen in the air and the susceptibility of the individual. Medical treatment generally aims to suppress the effects of pollen on the body cells; sufferers would rather not be susceptible at all.

The aim of this book is to give *all* hay fever sufferers the best possible chance of avoiding it. We believe that for the majority, perhaps as many as 80%, the suffering could be reduced to the level of a mere inconvenience. A fortunate 10% could be totally free of the condition. But we acknowledge that it is one of those unpalatable facts of life that for a minority, the symptoms will remain intractable. The unfortunate few many be stuck with hay fever unless it disappears spontaneously.

The first step in dealing with any problem is to understand it. We shall therefore explain the background to the disease, its causes, the way it produces its effects on sufferers, and the various methods of controlling or avoiding it. Once each person understands how his or her particular version of hay fever works, there is a much better chance of taking appropriate [preventive] action.

Successful treatment may involve the use of drugs or other types of therapy, or the avoidance of specific triggers, or a combination of strategies. Whatever course of action is chosen, half the battle with hay fever is to understand what is happening well enough to assist the body in the struggle against this unwanted condition. With any disease, attitudes to the problem and its treatment are important determinants of the degree to which sufferers are incapacitated by it.

This is not to imply that hay fever is 'all in the mind'. Far from it. We believe that hay fever could in fact be much more serious than has previously been recognised, because it is itself a symptom of larger problems in the world around us. Understanding this link between individual suffering and wider issues could enable us to deal more effectively with the causes and protect future generations from the continuing spread of the disease.

Surprising as it may seem to today's millions of hay fever

sufferers, the condition was practically unknown until the late nineteenth century. It was first reported in England, where Dr Blackley, who suffered from the disease, conducted the earliest systematic research on it. He commented in 1880: 'On the Continent, some [medical men] have never even heard of the disease'.

Looking for the reason behind this, some commentators have pointed to the parallel rise of the motor car, with its internal combustion engine expelling a cocktail of pollutants into the air for us to breathe. However, the answer is not so simple — although it is true that breathing exhaust fumes tends to make us more susceptible to allergic reactions.

How important each type of pollutant might be is one of the many unanswered questions about hay fever. Despite the prevalence of the condition, it is not a popular research topic. Besides, hay fever has several inconvenient features. It is not a problem that lends itself to easy investigation; it is too variable, fluctuating from day to day and even from hour to hour. Such variability means that researchers cannot get the sort of clear-cut results they like. Inconclusive results are not good for academic reputations.

Its early association with hay-making gave hay fever its name. But we now recognise that it is not drying hay, but the pollens from flowering grass, that produce the typical reaction in most sufferers. It can also be set off by pollens from trees, shrubs, and other flowers, and even the spores of some fungi. Whilst the peak season for the problem is the early summer, with 83% of sufferers reporting symptoms in June, some people will have hay fever at any time from late February to October.

Over the past hundred years, the pattern of the disease has changed. We have become allergic to a wider range of pollens, allergies have become more common, and the nature of the condition also seems to have changed.

Seasoned field workers at the turn of the century might have been amused to watch the adolescent farm hand caught in a sneezing fit. He would have been incapacitated for a couple of days or so — just long enough to avoid the hard work of getting in the hay. Town dwellers were not affected. Now, hay fever is more common in the city than in the country. It seems to be becoming a universal ailment.

Whereas the squire or farmer could perhaps afford to have his

17

lad off work for a day or two, the direct cost to the nation now is astronomical. Even though most hay fever sufferers struggle on, trying to maintain a normal working life despite their illness, four million working days are estimated to be lost each year because of hay fever.

What is at the heart of this expensive and distressing problem? It is an interaction that appears simple. Pollen grains inhaled with air get caught on moist membranes in the nose, throat, and in the eyes and ears, and stimulate the surface cells. In susceptible people these cells react, producing inflammation and soreness.

Once this reaction has begun, the whole system becomes sensitised. In this state an increasing number of substances will initiate and maintain the hay fever reaction.

At the height of the hay fever season, sufferers are liable to react badly to anything that smells of plants, or that looks like pollen in the air. Eyes water and swell and throats itch in response to perfumes that would have no ill-effects in the winter. Psychologists have found that people who suffer from severe hay fever will react to pictures of flowering grass in a totally pollen free room!

Next time you are in a cinema on a rainy summer day, listen for the sneezes that accompany a change of scene from indoors to a field or garden.

What then is pollen, and why should we react to it? Pollen is the plant equivalent of sperm, and it is produced by all flowering plants. When a plant is ready to reproduce, the first stage is to get a grain of pollen from the stamen of the male flower to the ovule of the female flower. There they fuse and grow to produce a seed.

Because plants cannot move, they generally go for massive numbers of seeds, some of which will stand a chance of being carried or scattered to fresh fertile ground. To produce all these seeds, flowers generally have many heads, and most plants too have many flowers. The number of pollen grains produced to achieve pollination defies the imagination. Only a microscopically small proportion of those produced will be successful in reaching the female plant, and from the fertile seeds produced only a very small number will grow to be mature plants, able once more to reproduce themselves.

We rely on a part of this incredibly productive cycle for our food supply. We take the bounty of seed produced before it is scattered, and in return nurture and protect the plants. Anyone who has looked over a wheat field ready for harvest, or grown peas or beans in a garden, will know just how prolific that bounty can be. We harvest an astonishing mountain of seed from plants.

Although the pollens most commonly responsible for hay fever are *not* those belonging to our food crops, the way we farm those crops may underlie the problem of the hay fever sufferer. It may be that modern agricultural methods have put stress on our old established wild grasses, weeds, and trees, which has provoked them into increasing their chances of reproducing.

Tests on hay fever sufferers reveal that they are most likely to be allergic to the wild or cultivated grasses that grow most profusely in their own locality.

In England the usual culprits are timothy grass, said to be the most potent allergen, and rye grass, which makes up something like 95% of the cultivated grass in farmers' fields in some areas. These are followed by species such as meadow grass, bent grass, fescues, and Yorkshire Fog.

Weeds also cause problems, especially American ragweed, which brings misery to thousands on the West Coast of both America and Canada. This plant has moved across the Atlantic, and is now colonising Britain, so it will probably crop up in our lists of allergens in the future. Troublesome native weeds include plantain, wormwood, mugwort and nettles.

Trees are the next major group of pollen allergen producers. The most usual sources are birch, plane, elder (whose flowers and berries make very good wine), poplar, and hazel. Finally, fungi, growing on organic materials, release spores to which some hay fever sufferers react. Although not the same as pollens, spores can have the same adverse effects, and everything we say about the way pollens produce their effects on us applies to spores as well.

These lists are far from complete. A very wide range of plant species can be implicated in any particular case. (See Appendices I, II, V, VI.)

But why should these apparently innocuous plants figure in the list of producers of triggering pollens? They are, after all, not new or overwhelming, they are not recently developed products of sophisticated human plant technology. We should have learned to live with their pollens generations ago. Yet the opposite seems to be true; we are becoming more sensitive to them each year.

A clue to the nature of the hay fever problem may lie in the very fact that these plants *are* old and well-established. We believe that it is quite possible that the increase in hay fever is associated with man's continued interference with the natural habitat of these plants. With each successive year, more land is drained and cleared for building or intensive agriculture, and the amount of space available for occupation by plants is decreased.

Not only are we limiting their habitat, we are interfering with the life-cycles of cultivated grasses by mowing or cutting them for silage before they can flower.

Like other living creatures under threat, plants will respond by trying to re-establish their numbers. Unlike animals, which may refrain from breeding until they move to a more congenial environment, plants, being unable to move, will need to produce more pollen to ensure their survival.

It may be that the millions of people who suffer from hay fever each year are paying the price for the increasingly specialised use of every part of the land in over-crowded countries. We have always tended to assume that plants are passive and, with a few exceptions, harmless. But it is just possible that the pressure of human demands on plant life has forced them to react in the only way they can, and increasing numbers of us are suffering as a result.

Humans have got where they are today by their ability to solve problems. If our view of the cause of this problem is correct, the final answer to hay fever would involve either eliminating the plants entirely, or de-stressing them to reduce their pollen levels. While the former course of action may have strong appeal to sufferers while under attack, it is obviously undesirable, if not impractical. The earth needs all its life-forms.

It is theoretically feasible to de-stress plants so that they can breed without massively increasing pollen production. The problem is that, as with so many other aspects of our natural environment that we have exploited without thought, we know too little about the requirements of an unstressed plant in terms of its ideal ecology.

A solution might involve creating carefully balanced plant reserves — parks, if you like — which are designed to create perfect conditions for the plants living in them. The rest of the country could then be devoted to agriculture.

Another possibility would be to plan the environment on a larger scale, taking account of the needs of all the lifeforms that co-exist. Wide strips of 'greenway' running across the countryside could be created as uninterrupted nature reserve, from which humans need not be excluded. Instead of bemoaning the loss of little hedgerows, we should admit that they have outlived their medieval purpose for man and replace them with megarows that would satisfy a diversity of needs for all the species that share the earth.

At the same time, the reduction of air and general pollution by the products of our technology is a health priority because of its importance not only to hay fever sufferers but to many others too.

Until a satisfactory solution can be found for all the protagonists involved, we have to apply our ingenuity and understanding in a variety of ways to cope with the hay fever problem.

The principle thrust of the modern attack on hay fever has involved the use of drugs. The object has been to find chemicals capable of suppressing the various symptoms of sensitivity to pollens. The drugs used generally block some part of the process involved at the molecular level.

The problem here is that many of the processes which produce the unwanted symptoms are also part of our normal everyday bodily activity. Drug action is unselective; if you block a process where it is not wanted, you will also block it where it is advantageous.

The latest range of anti-allergic drugs, used mainly for asthma, but also proving valuable for some hay fever sufferers, largely avoids this difficulty by relying on local application to the affected membranes. This reduces the side-effect problem considerably. However, these products do not reach inaccessible membranes, and they must be used before an attack starts and used continually until the danger of an attack is over. Once the sufferer is aware of the symptoms, it is too late to treat them.

The less than satisfactory treatments offered by drugs has led to the development of a variety of popular efforts at preventing symptoms. These range from the advocacy, by some doctors, of vaseline smeared round the nose, to the development of space

21

helmets like upside down goldfish bowls into which filtered air is pumped from a backpack.

The final major form of intervention used in the attempt to deal with hay fever is de-sensitisation (or hyposensitisation). It is a procedure that must be carried out well outside the hay fever season. The theory is that the body can become accustomed to pollens through the controlled administration of gradually increasing doses, so that it does not react when they appear in the air.

Conventional de-sensitisation begins with a series of skin tests, pricking the skin with various pollens to discover which ones cause a local reaction. Using this information, a cocktail of pollens is selected for injection into the sufferer. The treatment is usually repeated on three occasions, but it may take as many as eighteen injections, a week apart.

This works for some people, but it has serious drawbacks. It is a hazardous procedure which can result in death unless crucial precautions are taken.

The hay fever sufferer has to weigh the risks against the likely benefits of each type of medical treatment. These are described in detail in Chapter Five.

For some hay fever sufferers, a miracle will happen. One year, just as the disease came to them out of the blue, it will leave them again. They will be free of it. The reasons for this spontaneous remission may be as idiosyncratic as the cause of the condition, but because they are not known, there is no certain way of hastening the process.

We have become accustomed to believing that modern medicine has answers to most of our health problems. But this belief does not stand up to scrutiny. While the mechanical arts, such as surgery and bone-setting, and replacement therapies like the use of insulin in diabetes, are generally successful, the results are not so dramatic in the less clear-cut areas of medicine. Life-limiting conditions can rumble on inconclusively for years.

This is definitely true of hay fever. There has been no claim for a marvellous breakthrough in research which might bring new hope to hay fever sufferers. This may be because the drug manufacturers, those vastly profitable multinational companies which fund most medical research, cannot see sufficient profit in a very seasonal market. Whether or not their efforts would in any case

22

be more successful in hay fever treatment than they have been in others, such as the massive arthritis market, is debateable.

The majority of hay fever sufferers find only incomplete relief from conventional medicine. Most of those who rely on drugs express some degree of dissatisfaction with their treatment.

What is needed is a combination of approaches that can be tailored to suit each individual, giving the maximum benefit with the minimum of risk and unwanted side-effects. To achieve this, we have to reverse the usual approach to hay fever. Instead of looking at the sneeze, or the swollen eyes, and trying to stop these localised symptoms with local measures, we should step right back. We need to be far enough away to look at the individual and the environment. We must broaden our view of the possible solutions.

Sometimes the cause of the disease can be disconnected from the life of the potential sufferer. The first and most obvious course of action, from this perspective, would be for the sufferer to consider moving away from an area where there is a high level of pollution, or where the problem pollens are common, to a place where both are absent, or at least considerably less common. This may seem drastic, but for some long-term chronic victims it could be the only answer.

Although de-sensitisation is an attractive idea, as generally practised it has a poor success record. But the approach adopted by some homoeopathic doctors does seem to be on the right track. It involves the administration of infinitesimally small doses of the triggering pollens. In this way, they aim to gently persuade the body to accept pollen with imperceptible reaction. The great advantage of this approach is that it is absolutely safe.

It may be some time before the full benefits of a progressive approach to disconnecting sufferers from the effects of triggers become apparent. Immediate results cannot usually be expected. Hay fever does not begin in an instant, so any cure is most unlikely to be instant.

What usually happens is that the body becomes gradually more and more pressured into over-reaction to a particular pollen. When this susceptibility reaches a certain point, something allows the triggering reaction to start. The experience of immigrants to North America suggests that the whole process takes between three and five years for most people; after this period, those who are susceptible will show the symptoms of ragweed pollen allergy.

So, in the search for a complete cure, the removal or reduction of the final trigger should be regarded merely as the first step. The long-term aim should be the reduction of the pressures which produce allergic reactions. This will provide a margin of safety beyond just being free from the obvious symptoms of hay fever.

Does this approach work? In recent years, more people have been prepared to take a wider look at their annual misery. The publicity given to environmental factors involved in cases of total allergy syndrome have prompted second thoughts about the wisdom of simply stopping the sneezing and leaving it at that. Many have found that if they are prepared to think in terms of a two or three year approach to reducing allergic susceptibility to the barest minimum, then they will no longer have a problem with hay fever.

We can say this with absolute confidence. One of us used to be one of the most irritable, miserable, unhappy and unlivable-with incapacitated hay fever sufferers you are ever likely to have been unfortunate enough to meet.

Dark rooms and damp towels in summer, falling asleep on too many drugs, persistant sore throats, feeling over-heated, swollen eyes, and a deep resentful aversion to any of the joys of spring or summer was his lot from the age of fourteen to forty-one.

After three years of treatment, the story is totally different.

A permanent love affair has developed between Colin and the summer. It embraces all the signs of that time of year, from the greening of the spring meadows and leaf buds emerging on trees to the blooming of the flowers.

Hay fever is such a minimal problem that sport is once more on the calendar, and running through the night scented summer air is a positively intoxicating delight.

This pleasure can overwhelm innocent bystanders. They get dragged away from whatever they are doing and pressganged into sharing the pleasure of breathing some long-forgotten perfume from shrub or flower, recalling dim memories of misspent youth.

The near-total cure was a most joyous discovery. The freedom to be and enjoy all life's experiences once more is something beyond the power of description.

It is our hope that all hay fever sufferers will be able to recover their share of the appreciation of the natural world. Particularly those parts of that nature that may at present be regarded as implacable enemies.

2 The size of the problem

Every year in Britain approximately *eight million* people suffer from hay fever badly enough to seek medication for their symptoms.

The disease is so widespread that it is the only condition for which daily bulletins, in the form of pollen counts or pollen predictions, are issued on the radio and TV. Throughout the summer months many people listen for the pollen count in the hope that perhaps tomorrow their symptoms might not be so bad, or to enable them to adjust the quantity of drugs they will take in the attempt to beat those symptoms. Some sufferers use the pollen and weather forecasts to decide whether they will go out or not. For most people with hay fever, the pollen count is a generalised predictor of misery.

In the western industrialised countries, which like Britain have a temperate climate, between 10% and 15% of the entire population will suffer from hay fever. In America and Europe that amounts to over 100 million ruined summers.

Once spring has stirred the plants into flowering it is simply a matter of time before the familiar symptoms begin. And every year will bring a new crop of people who are experiencing the misery of hay fever for the first time.

Before considering the symptoms that allow the diagnosis of hay fever, perhaps we should deal with one myth, or more correctly, a misnomer. Fever, in the true medical sense, is not a symptom or a part of the condition. Hay fever was a good enough description at the time when the disease was first identified. Later, when knowledge of the subject increased, it was realised that the description was technically wrong, but by then it was too late to change it.

What sufferers may feel is a localised overheating of the skin,

26

particularly around the face and neck, with a reddening similar to blushing. This response is fairly common in young children and adolescents who suffer from the disease. The fever is more a feeling than a fact.

For all that, the sensation is real enough for the sufferer, as are all the other symptoms. They emerge with the flowers from their annual hibernation, ending that blissful period of snuffle-free normality and free breathing that makes hay fever sufferers welcome the clear air and frosts of winter.

The defining characteristic of hay fever is the seasonal occurrence of the same pattern of symptoms. At first, they may be mild: an annoying buzzing or ringing in the ears, usually accompanied by itching eyes and mouth. Next in the escalating array of symptoms are those usually associated with the common cold: running nose, sore throat, and sneezing fits that can become infuriating.

Then come the more serious symptoms. Most hay fever sufferers experience only a few, if any, of these, but a very high pollen count means that the numbers inevitably rise.

Contact between pollen grains and the hypersensitive surface of the eye can result in sore, discharging eyes (vernal catarrh). Sometimes, the tissues of the face around the eyes will swell to frog-like proportions. The eyelids can become swollen and inflamed, and in severe cases the delicate membrane covering the inside of the eyelid and the eye itself — the conjunctiva — may develop surface lumps aptly named 'cobblestone papillae'. Rubbing on the front of the eye, these occasionally lead to ulceration and permanent damage to vision.

As if this were not enough, the nose, which began by itching, also becomes swollen, dripping constantly or blocking up. Sometimes, polyps form on the engorged tissue in the nose, narrowing the nostril further. The inflammation spreads to the sinuses, the eustachian tubes which connect the throat with the ear, and down the throat to the bronchi. All these tubes and cavities can gum up with mucus. The sneeze changes to a cough, perhaps producing globs of sputum. Breathing becomes still more difficult.

Some people develop asthma as the muscles round the air-tubes to the lungs go into spasm, but non-asthmatics will also wheeze. This adds to the difficulty of coughing up mucus, which may accumulate, exacerbating the problem.

While few hay fever sufferers are totally incapacitated by their symptoms for more than short periods each season, the majority find that they can be bad enough at times to lead them to total despair. The thought that every summer can be ruined by misery that continues for weeks and months together, and that relief from the dark, dank British winter will be denied is a recipe for depression.

While others enjoy the long sun-filled days and balmy evenings, the hay fever sufferer will be preoccupied with searching out cool, pollen free places, a box of tissues in hand.

Hay fever is in every sense a life-limiting condition. Not only does it restrict the leisure options of the individual for a significant part of the year, but it also affects job opportunities and performance in the sufferer's career. Nobody can be expected to excel during months when they are suffering the symptoms of hay fever, or when coping with the unwanted effects of medicines aimed at suppressing these symptoms.

Unfortunately for hay fever sufferers, almost all the major examinations in England, Wales and Northern Ireland which can determine future prospects coincide with the pollen season. University finals, for example, are taken in June. So are the qualifying school and college examinations, as well as most of the trade examinations. The academic year is structured in a way which is bound to pose problems for the victims of hay fever.

Research into the effects on performance has demonstrated the importance of this problem.

One study showed that hay fever sufferers were significantly less accurate in a task where they worked under time pressure. Surprisingly, perhaps, they were as fast as their more fortunate fellows; but success in crucial tasks like examinations demands precision too.

A door-to-door survey carried out for Merrell Pharmaceuticals revealed that over a quarter of hay fever sufferers are students. Half of these reported that hay fever or the side-effects of treatment for the condition had adverse effects on their work.

In a second survey, carried out in schools and universities, it was found that hay fever beginning early in life (below age six) was twice as common among 'O' level candidates as it was among 'A' level and degree candidates. The implication of this is that hay fever may affect 'O' level results so seriously that many sufferers never pass this first hurdle and consequently do not achieve the career of which they might otherwise be capable.

Some of the comments made by the students surveyed clearly reveal their individual misery.

Here are examples:

'I feel extremely tired during the day and find concentration is extremely limited. My eyes are continuously blurred and my nose is either running or blocked.'

'Unable to wear contact lenses due to watery eyes, therefore unable to see the work.'

'I did not feel like doing anything at all. I was affected pretty bad during "A" level exams.'

'Having to carry around "drug store" and boxes of tissues and eye drops — physical appearance pretty gruesome during hay fever season.'

'It is a bit difficult taking notes and studying when your nose is continually running and your eyes are sore/red and you are sneezing nonstop.'

When the illness is at its worst, work can become impossible. The individual who chooses, or has been trained, to work outdoors surrounded by the plants to which he or she develops an allergy may be forced to give up the job. The sportsperson whose passion is to play tennis or cricket or any outdoor game at the height of the summer may face the loss of a much-valued activity. And even the city office-worker may have to stay at home in a cool, dark bedroom because swollen eyes or an uncontrollably dripping nose make work impossible.

Unfortunately, the effects of the condition are not confined to the individual. It is perhaps little wonder that with symptoms of this nature, which produce a sense of being cheated of the summers of the sufferer's life, will lead to a certain amount of irritability.

Disturbed sleep and continued discomfort must also take their toll. This can vary from mild edginess to utterly impossible behaviour, as everyone who has lived with a hay fever sufferer will know.

This is one woman's experience of her second husband's illness:

'Living with him, I found myself wondering whether it would not be wise to ask potential partners whether they suffered from hay fever *before* falling in love! I'd met him at the end of August, and it hadn't occurred to me that I might have to put up with the same summer miseries as I'd known with the last one. But you can't reject someone when he's utterly unloveable for the best part of three months every year because of illness, can you?

'But the truth is, hay fever limited our lives quite severely. I'm a sun worshipper; I adore the hot days of June and July, and I want to be out there, playing in the grass, going for long walks, enjoying the summer every way I can. How can you enjoy it, though, when your partner is complaining all the time, and demands to be driven home early when you've just gone out for a picnic?

'The children, too, missed out. His youngest daughter well remembers the time he took the boys riding cross-country on the back of his motorbike — and then when her turn came round, he couldn't do it any more because his eyes were too swollen. That sort of thing happened again and again.

'He just didn't have the energy to do anything. His work-rate went right down, and being self-employed, that meant that there were potentially serious financial consequences. And that knowledge, of course, added to our difficulties. We had money problems to cope with on top of everything else for many years.

'Finally I decided I would take my summer holiday without him, so we didn't both get dragged down by his hay fever. I was going to go away with my sister in June. But the guilt, of course, held me back — you can't feel comfortable about leaving somebody to be ill on his own. Thankfully, that was the year he found the answer.

'There were things we could have done about it, mind. I know that now. But he was so angry at having hay fever at all, he just resented it and assumed that when doctors couldn't help much, there wouldn't be anything we could do.

'He'd tried the usual medical approaches, naturally. He used to get through so many antihistamine tablets, he'd fall asleep in the afternoons and wake up more irritable than ever when the effects wore off. Nothing else worked at all. As for desensitisation, he was ill for ten days after the first injection, so he didn't go for any more.

'For my part, well, I thought he'd gone into it all thoroughly, and I couldn't do anything to help except try to make him comfortable, which was impossible. If only we'd known what we know now! We could have avoided so much suffering.'

Some of that must sound all too familiar to many long-standing hay fever sufferers and their families.

At times, the imposition of an otherwise fairly innocuous domestic burden will prove too much, the last straw for the simmering sufferer, inducing an uncharacteristic and unreasonable outburst of shouting or even physical violence. Typically this is seen as an irrational act, a burst of temper which is over as quickly as it began. The perpetrator feels some slight relief, but this is masked by the remorse which follows. The hay fever victim ends up still more miserable, and the unhappiness of the condition is spread among those nearest and most vulnerable.

While adults may be able to rationalise outbursts of this sort and achieve some reconciliation based on understanding, it is likely to be more complicated when children are involved. Unless parents are aware of the reason for it, a seemingly unwarranted episode of bad or violent behaviour may be put down to wickedness and punished.

All ill health tends to make the best of us crotchety at times, and a subtle condition, waxing and waning as hay fever does, is no exception. In fact, as we shall see later, the complex chemical processes that occur in the bodies of sufferers are quite capable of provoking bouts of nastiness.

Is it possible to draw a picture of the typical sufferer?

Although hay fever is not one of those diseases that strikes at a single clearly-defined sector of the population, some groups are particularly at risk.

Women are slightly more susceptible than men, and young people are much more susceptible than their parents.

Those who are born just before, or during the hay fever season are more likely to develop the illness. In Finland, where birch pollen allergy is common, it has been estimated that the incidence of the disease could be reduced by 28% if hay fever sufferers would avoid having children in the months when the pollen count is high!

General anaesthetics given to babies and toddlers of less than two years old are also associated with a higher risk of hay fever in later life, possibly because of damage to the respiratory tract.

Repeated respiratory infections seem to have a similar effect.

Most people who have allergic problems live in cities. The highest concentration of hay fever victims are in those cities that are surrounded by high populations of the most allergenic plants. The worst place in the world to live seems to be one of the cities in the North-East of the United States. There the incidence of hay fever among college students can be as high as 25%.

Most sufferers experience their first bout of hay fever in their early teens. The age at which the prevalence of the disease reaches its maximum is around fifteen. The condition often seems to develop with the complex changes involved in reaching maturity, but it can occur for the first time in people of almost any age. It is very rare however for babies to be afflicted, and almost equally rare that an elderly person will suddenly develop it for the first time.

In other cases the specific allergy to pollen may be one of a series of related problems. A generalised tendency to suffer this type of reaction can be signalled by childhood eczema, followed by adolescent onset of hay fever, and finally food allergy or asthma in middle to late life.

To the great disappointment of some who thought themselves to be ex-hay fever victims, spontaneous remission is not always permanent. Not only can allergic symptoms return in a slightly altered form, but hay fever itself can start up again after a temporary disappearance. Individual susceptibility normally varies from year to year, and the environmental conditions which precipitate hay fever also vary, both from season to season, and from day to day in any particular summer. The interaction of these influences means that the course of the disease can be very erratic.

It is easier to predict which individuals are most likely to suffer from hay fever on the basis of their own and their familial medical history. They are the young people who have experienced outbreaks of eczema or asthma, or who have close relatives who suffer from allergies.

Four out of five hay fever sufferers have a family history of allergy. Of those who do not suffer from the condition, only one in three has a close relative who does.

Some geneticists believe that the level of the crucial substance in the body that is implicated in the production of allergic responses (IgE: its significance will be explained in chapter 3) is determined by the genes we inherit from our parents.

However, the family relationships are not straightforward because this is a condition where different genes interact with one another to produce the total picture, and there are strong environmental influences. All we inherit is a generalised *tendency* to react, or not to react, to potential allergens.

What geneticists cannot explain when they estimate the inheritability of hay fever is why the problem is so much more widespread today than it was a hundred years ago — when our great-grandparents, whose genetic makeup we have inherited, were alive. Then, it was still quite rare, and thought to be primarily a problem of the 'educated classes', maybe because those who wrote and spoke about it tended to be doctors who suffered from the condition themselves.

The first description of hay fever was given by just such an individual. In 1819, Dr John Bostock read a paper in London on a 'Case of a Periodical Affection of the Eyes and Chest'. After this initial paper, he received 'distinct accounts of eighteen cases', and ten others in which 'the accounts were less perfect'. Even in 1854, a Dr Walshe maintained that 'The complaint occurs only at the periods of hay-making, or when the odour of grass is powerful, and is of exceedingly rare occurrence'.

Precisely how common it is now is hard to determine. Adequate surveys of large populations have not been carried out. Estimates vary from the figure of 8% of the people of the USA, and 25% of the students of some American colleges, to 1.2% of the patients attending a North London G.P.

More reliable British figures are those from a door-to-door survey of 1,210 representative households. It found that one household in five included at least one person who had suffered from hay fever the previous summer. Extrapolating these results to the country as a whole, this means that over nine million people had hay fever in 1981. This was a year in which the pollen count was exceptionally low.

The average G.P. will see between five and ten people with hay fever every day in the peak month of June, but many of those who have mild forms of the condition, or who recognise it from family experience, will deal with it themselves and not seek a doctor's help. These people will never show up in any medical statistics. In a typical year, only around half of those who suffer from hay fever will consult a doctor about it, although most of the others will have done so at some time.

Many do not consult their G.P.s because they feel that doctors do not take the condition sufficiently seriously. But this is less likely to be true of hay fever than of the less clear-cut allergies; sufferers from these have often been classified as neurotic attention-seekers.

In addition to the identified sufferers, there is an unknown number of hidden sufferers, including those who have some of the typical features of the condition but not the full range. During childhood, especially, the runny nose and sneezes may be put down to summer colds.

Other hidden sufferers may not be able to tell the difference between the common cold and hay fever. In high pollen years it is noticeable that many more people complain of summer colds or even influenza, than in low pollen summers. It is quite feasible that a sizeable proportion of these people are suffering from hay fever, perhaps for the first time, as the pollen level or type breaches their threshold and they become allergic.

Hidden sufferers are part of the hay fever picture that is inevitably blurred. The symptoms that are commonly associated with the condition become less distinct with marginal sufferers.

In addition to this, the underlying cause of hay fever can give rise to other symptoms which are so distinct and obvious that they are classed as separate diseases in their own right.

Among them are eczema, hives, and asthma. Highly susceptible invididuals tend to suffer from a combination of these conditions, with one being the dominant complaint and the others following in its wake. In their turn, these conditions may bring further minor general symptoms such as rashes, headaches, abdominal cramps and diarrhoea.

This spread of symptoms, from the particular ones which are the accepted indicators of hay fever, to the more general ones, leads us to a position where we can place hay fever in its context. The common mechanism that underlies all these symptoms is that of the allergic response.

The condition we call hay fever is a particular sort of allergic reaction. The exact nature of this reaction for hay fever sufferers will be explained in the next chapter, but in order to get to grips with the size of the hay fever problem we first need to have a general picture of allergies; what they are; what causes them; how common they are, and how serious they can be.

The *Encyclopaedia Britannica* defines an allergy as the 'exaggerated reactivity to foreign substances that sometimes occurs following exposure to those substances'. In simple terms being allergic to something means that it will upset you in some way.

The whole question of allergies is a fairly new one in medical literature. The word allergy was first suggested by a Frenchman, Clemens von Pirquet, in 1906. He used it as a term to cover all changes in reactivity that could be caused in human patients, and in animals. Since that time the word has come to be used to describe only *increased* reactivity. And it has also become usual to describe someone as being allergic to some specific thing.

Allergic reactions were first identified in medicine with the growth of immunisation as a means of protecting people against infectious diseases. The vaccines used were made by infecting animals, or a suitable animal product culture, with a specific disease organism. When the disease organism, usually a virus, had multiplied in the host or the culture, they were extracted and killed, or 'attenuated', so that they were harmless.

The mixture would then be injected into the person to be immunised. The harmless dead viruses would fool the body into reacting as if they were alive. It would go into a defensive routine that would enable it to resist a real attack by live viruses of the same disease at a later time.

Unfortunately some people were upset by the protein molecules from the culture or animals' blood that remained in the injection. They suffered an exaggerated reactivity to these foreign substances.

As more was discovered about the immune system, it was realised that allergic reactions occurred because the body treated whatever it was reacting against as a dangerous invader, and the appropriate part of the immune system attempted to deal with them. The problem was that, compared to the numbers encountered in nature there were so many of them entering the body at the same time, that severe problems were caused to the body in question.

Since that time, allergic reactions have come to be associated with a wide range of substances. Their initial association with

35

foreign proteins has widened to include reactions to common foods and the whole range of artificial chemicals that are now present in every part of our lives.

Nevertheless, the basis of all these unwanted reactions is the same. The body reacts to a foreign protein or strange chemicals which it treats as a threat.

Most of our reactions to proteins are entirely benign. When we eat them as an essential part of our food, they are good for us; our digestive systems break them down to be rebuilt into the tissues of our bodies. Usually we are unaware of the proteins surrounding us in the biosphere. They can in no way be regarded as dangerous substances.

Proteins have been called 'the stuff of life'. Not a single living organism, no matter whether microscopic or enormous, plant or animal, has been found that does not contain protein molecules in every part of it. Proteins are very large molecules, made up of thousands of atoms, and their peculiar characteristic is that they twist themselves up into highly complicated shapes.

The thousands of atoms of which the proteins are made are themselves formed into sub-units called amino acids. These are the building blocks from which all proteins are made. There are twenty-two different sorts of amino acid, and they can combine in almost any sequence, so the number of possible varieties of protein molecule is almost infinite. (Twenty-two multiplied by twenty-two, twenty-two times.)

Every living organism can be described in terms of the various sorts of protein of which it is made up. This is a very precise process; even humans, who are roughly all the same, have to be careful to cross-match their blood before transfusions. If you were to compare the proteins in a human with those in a chimpanzee, you would find less then 1% which were different, yet the difference between the two species is obvious.

Individuals within the same species, you and me for instance, have minute yet crucial differences in the proteins of which we are made. It may be regarded as nothing short of miraculous that each body can recognise its own combination of proteins making up all its individual tissues and organs, and accept them, while rejecting absolutely those essentially similar proteins that it would encounter in somebody else's kidney.

Overcoming these defences is one of the major problems for

transplant surgery, and the reason for the enormous trouble taken to match the tissues of organ donor and recipient. Despite the careful match, the body will attempt to reject any organ unless it comes from an identical twin who shares precisely the same protein pattern. The worse the tissue match, the more rapid and severe will be the rejection, and the defence mechanisms will escalate their action into a fight to the death if necessary, to overcome the intruder. This automatic reaction to the presence of foreign proteins has to be suppressed indefinitely with powerful and dangerous drugs if a transplant is to succeed.

Most life forms have some sort of defence against foreign proteins. The more developed the life form, the more complex and sophisticated this defence is likely to be. In the simple bacteria, the mechanism takes the form of molecular manipulation. Bacteria resistant to penicillin, for example, have learned to produce a substance that causes the penicillin molecule to fall apart so that they cannot be affected by it. Simple single celled creatures tend to swallow enemies, and then take them apart, keeping the useful bits and rejecting the rest.

Humans have many levels of defence, and more defence in depth within the various levels. We have bacteria in our guts which act as chemical engineers in our digestive processes, and we also have single celled defenders in our blood, white cells which engulf any invaders they may encounter. In addition, we have a range of immune mechanisms that produce a variety of counter measures to invasion by infectious organisms, poisons, or the mechanical damage caused by the fracture of a limb or a bite.

Hay fever is rarely a life-or-death struggle. It develops when one level of the immune defence options is wrongly triggered into action by a harmless protein, and will not acknowledge the error. This is the allergic response.

It is a measure of the complexity of humans and their defence systems, that although allergic reactions have been identified for some time, and although many theories have been put forward to explain their precise causes and the reasons for the symptoms that are provoked, no single approach covers all the phenomena that have been recorded.

With such complexity, it is not surprising that there are many degrees of seriousness of allergic reactions. It was the most

37

serious of these that first brought the subject into prominence: death from anaphylactic shock.

Approximately twenty people die each year in Britain from anaphylactic shock caused by sensitivity to penicillin. That is why you should always be asked if you are allergic to it before being given a penicillin injection, and why you should inform your doctor if you develop a skin rash — often the first warning of allergy — when taking penicillin.

Perhaps anaphylactic shock is best thought of as the consequence of a complicated and sophisticated system being pushed just a little too far. In an anaphylactic reaction, a local part of the body swells up and becomes congested with fluid. This may be the best way to localise a dose of a foreign or poisonous substance, so that the body can deal with it without it spreading. But when overwhelming quantities of substances capable of causing such a reaction are injected into the body, it cannot localise the problem.

Death from anaphylactic shock is very rare in nature. The most probable circumstances would occur when a unusually sensitive individual is stung by insects, and over-reacts to the poison injected. But it is hard to see why the body should have developed a protective system which has the capacity to go so badly wrong that insect bites can be fatal.

This is why it was only noticed when immunisation using animal serum became widespread. Once a large quantity of foreign protein had been injected deep into the patient's tissues, little could be done to prevent the devastating reaction that sometimes followed.

The most recent development in the allergy story has been the emergence of what has come to be called 'total allergy syndrome'. In this condition, people are described as being allergic to the twentieth century, because they react badly to artificial materials such as plastics, synthetic fabrics, paints, and so on. The only treatment that seems to offer any benefit is to place sufferers in an environment that contains no such substances.

Even their food must be carefully selected and prepared so that sufferers can avoid eating any of the many preservatives, colourings, artificial flavourings or sweeteners which most foods contain today. It is a serious problem for those who become so afflicted. Fortunately, only a small number of sufferers have so far been identified.

For most people who are aware of an allergy, the problem of

dealing with it is comparatively straightforward. Through experience they learn what substances they are allergic to, and they do their best to avoid them.

Food allergy has recently been recognised as a much bigger problem than was previously suspected, and many people have found that some long-term illness has disappeared with a change in eating habits. Allergy to cows' milk, for instance, is particularly common. It was intended for young cattle, after all.

Susceptibility to any allergic reaction is largely an individual matter. While one thing may affect you severely, it could leave thousands untouched. The range of substances to which individuals have been found to react includes almost any protein, many artificial chemicals, many natural substances taken in excessive quantities, and a wide variety of the products of our way of life.

The growing size of the problem has given birth to a new branch of medical science, that of *clinical ecology*. The concern that inspired the growth of this speciality was expressed in books such as *Our Synthetic Environment*, written by American Murray Bookchin in 1962, and followed by many popular works dealing with specific parts of the environmental problem, such as Rachel Carson's classic *Silent Spring*.

Clinical ecologists point to what amounts to a vast underswell of sub-clinical illness caused by the environmental deterioration to which we are all subjected. Sub-clinical illnesses are conditions which are just bad enough to detract from life, but not bad, or definite, enough to take effective action against.

They are typified by the generalised 'under the weather' feeling which seems to afflict more and more people for much of the time. It is a permanent listlessness and lack of vitality. A victim of this condition is particularly likely to fall victim to recognised clinical problems such as colds, 'flu and other infections, because it results in a general lowering of resistance.

The cause of this sub-clinical malaise is rooted in the steadily increasing use of artificial chemicals in every sphere of modern life. People who suffer these largely unrecognised conditions are the victims of chemical susceptibility.

It is generally accepted that certain industrial processes and chemicals can constitute health risks, with consequences ranging from mild rashes to cancer. One of the oldest man-made hazards came from the use of lead for water pipes, and one of many recent ones is the danger posed by the nuclear industry. Despite this long history, we have been slow to realise that the apparently good products of industry may also entail the possibility of widespread harm.

The realisation of the scale of this problem has only slowly come to light. When doctors decided to trace the cause of what came to be known as 'multiple fruit allergy', a typical chain of relationships was discovered. Sufferers from this allergy reacted badly to a wide range of fruits, but there seemed to be no obvious pattern. At first it was assumed that the solution would be simple; find the fruit that triggered the reaction, eliminate it from the diet, and all would be well.

But this approach was unsuccessful. The investigation widened to other possibilities and the solution to the problem was discovered. The 'fruit allergy' was not triggered by fruit at all, but by the supposedly harmless pesticides that were habitually sprayed on to apples.

Since then, a growing number of investigative trails have led research workers into the maze of man-made molecules to find the causes of particular complaints. The links between food colourings and hyperactivity in children are perhaps the best known example of this phenomenon.

Artificial chemicals that would not normally exist in nature have been put to use in every part of our lives. Our soil is drenched with them to wring more profit from agriculture, our industry eagerly substitutes them for more expensive natural resources, and we accept the convenience they bring to our lives. As a consequence, the food we eat, the water we drink, and the air we breathe, is unavoidably contaminated.

Under this environmental loading, we do what we are so good at doing: we adapt. Humans have been so successful at adapting to changes in the environment that we behave as if this ability had no limits. But clearly it has, and it is when we reach the limit of our personal capacity that we produce symptoms of the stress we are under.

Hay fever is just one of the ways these cumulative stress loadings can be triggered into a disease condition. The final straw is the foreign proteins of pollen. But it is likely that the reaction occurs when it does because of additional stress from other sources. These can include lifestyle changes, emotional stresses, bereavement or loss, or another apparently unconnected episodes of ill health.

It seems, however, that exposure to the particular types of chemicals associated with industrial development plays a crucial role in producing pollen-sensitive individuals. For although there are mentions of allergic reactions in history — even the ancient Greeks knew of their existence — they were very rare. And hay fever, as we have seen, was unknown. The growth of hay fever into the mass affliction of today is a phenomenon of the last two hundred years. Britain can, in fact, claim another first. The rise in hay fever parallels the spread of the industrial revolution.

Industrial pollution seems to have stirred up those body systems which contribute to the allergic response. In this alerted condition, those who are susceptible react much more readily to a wide range of substances. Today these range from house and pet dust, fur, mites and moulds, paint and fuel fumes to washing powders and potato peelings.

Hay fever sufferers are peculiar in that they experience a seasonal reaction triggered by plant pollens and spores. The season for airborne pollens starts in the spring with trees and shrubs, goes through the summer with grasses and other soft plants, and ends when the frosts stop the fungi spreading their spores.

Can we summarise the constituents of hay fever? Individual luck certainly plays a part, both in being susceptible and in failing to adapt to the stress of the background loading of allergens. The triggering of an identifiable reaction by plant pollens produces the visible symptoms of the condition.

This is accurate, but it may not be the complete picture. As we shall see in the next chapter the size of the hay fever problem may have a final twist that has not been considered before.

3   *What causes hay fever?*

The simple and most obvious answer is pollen.

Like most simple and obvious answers, this one is incomplete. Nevertheless, it provides a logical starting point in understanding hay fever.

Pollen is a powder-like substance produced by mature flowering plants. The name derives from Latin, and may be roughly translated as 'fine flour'. This is appropriate because pollen grains are very small, usually invisible to the naked eye, although easily seen with a good microscope. Their size is measured in microns; one micron is one thousandth of a millimetre. Most grains of pollen are between 5 and 200 microns in diameter and roughly spherical in shape.

Pollen is essential to pollination, the process by which plants produce fertile seeds. Each grain of pollen, like a human sperm, is a single cell containing the male half of the genetic material required to produce a fertile seed. When it is carried to the female half, which stays on the plant in the female flower, the two fuse and a growth process begins which ends with the production of seeds.

So to produce a fertile seed, the pollen grain has to get from the stamen, or male part of the flower that produces it, to the stigma, the reproductive part of the female flower. This is achieved by a variety of means, often not unconnected with the traditional activities of the bees, if not usually the birds.

The flowers that we tend to find attractive have evolved to appeal to insects. By attracting and feeding insects, the plants get them to carry their sticky pollens from one flower to another so that they can reproduce. Particular sorts of insects are attracted to particular features of flowers, their colours, perfumes, and shapes; for example, many butterflies are attracted to blue flowers, and night-flying moths are drawn to flowers which produce strong scents at nightfall.

Other plants achieve pollination by a variety of methods. Some use birds, animals, water and even slugs or snails. And of course the method that most concerns us, the release of pollen into the air. There it relies entirely on the chance action of the wind to carry it to a female flower of the same species.

One interesting feature of wind pollination is that, in evolutionary terms, it is a relatively recent development. Between twelve and three million years ago (which *is* recent in evolution!), the dense tropical and sub-tropical forests that covered much of the world were shrinking under the influence of global climatic change. As the plants thinned out into what was for them, though not for our ancestors, an increasingly hostile environment, so the chances of direct or short-range pollination decreased. Under these circumstances, more and more plant species came to rely on the vagaries of the wind for their survival.

Casting pollen to the wind is not as effective as having it delivered by insects. To compensate for this, the male flowers began to produce much more pollen. One weed which is common in cultivated land in southern England, *Mercurialis annua*, or annual mercury, has a male flower that produces 1,250 million grains of pollen.

Grasses are less prolific per flower, but they compensate for this by having many more flowers per plant. The pollen from annual mercury may not travel much further than a quarter of a mile or so, but the cumulative effect of all the plants which rely on wind pollination can ensure that there is more than enough pollen about, certainly as far as humans are concerned.

Naturally enough, some plants have become well adapted to wind pollination. The pollen grains of pine trees have air sacs that allow them to be carried up to five hundred miles from their starting-point without much difficulty. It is a spectacular, if slightly horrifying, sight to see the green haze of pollen rising in warm air over evergreen forests.

Wind-pollinated plants tend to have relatively long stems which expose their flowers high in the air and light. Common examples in Britain are the grasses, rushes and sedges, nettles and plantains, and hazel, birch, poplar, and oak. Under the right conditions for each particular plant, perhaps gusting wind or warmer than usual sunshine, the flowers burst open to scatter their pollen.

Different plants thrive under different conditions, living in balance with others sharing the same environment. Some wind pollinated plants like to grow in clumps on open ground, others as scattered individuals. They all have preferred patterns which are influenced by a range of factors. The more favourable the conditions, the better the plant will do.

Conditions in Britain favour a wide range of plants. Intensive use of the land produces a variety of mono-cultures, from the grain fields of East Anglia to the coniferous blight to which much of Wales, the north of England and Scotland are subjected.

It is perhaps unfortunate that our temperate zone climate, with its fairly wide extremes of summer and winter temperatures and countryside with a wide range of altitudes and local environments, may be better suited to wind pollinated plants than it is to humans.

Because of the way it is intended to work, each pollen grain is designed a bit like a space capsule. Inside, the male germ cell carries the genetic message in the nucleus, which is surrounded by granular nutritional material, all packaged in a thin inner coating. This is the vital cargo and its stores. It is relatively short lived, capable of surviving for only a few days. Around this inner core is a comparatively massive shell made of protein molecules bound together in a very tough structure. This protein shell is thick, lumpy, and impenetrable, designed to protect its precious contents.

The tough outer shell of the pollen grain is highly resistant to decay. Because of this, it has proved very useful to scientists investigating the plant life of the past; using intact pollen grains, they have been able to identify the specific plant families that were alive over a million years ago.

So accurate is the information from pollen grains that examination of samples from two and a half million years ago up to around ten thousand years ago shows the impact of climatic changes, such as the onset and retreat of the ice ages.

They also reveal the changes marking the time when the first human groups began to cultivate the soil instead of living a nomadic hunting and gathering existence. Around this time, some twenty thousand years ago, pollen profiles from northern

44

and central Europe show the appearance of pollens from cultivated cereal crops.

These pollen profiles are particularly important because they contain greatly increased amounts of pollen from plants that are now regarded as agricultural weeds. Our stone age ancestors cleared the temperate woodland by cutting and burning, much as primitive people still do today.

In cultivating the cleared land, Neolithic man did two things. He made it possible for more humans to survive on less land, and can thus be blamed for starting the population explosion. He also gave the same chance to those plants to which we appear to be particularly sensitive.

By settling to agriculture and foresaking the roaming life of the previous two or three million years, our Neolithic ancestors unwittingly initiated trends that resulted in the development of the disease of hay fever as we experience it today.

While humans were on the move, their impact on the environment was hardly more or less than that of the other animals. Once the age of settlement began, the fixed location, with its increasing numbers, put pressure on all the other life forms in the same area. It is a process that continues today. Satellites in space map and record every possible resource that humans can exploit. The needs of other inhabitants of the planet are overlooked in the scramble to fulfill the demand for 'more'.

At the beginning of this human pressure wave, or even perhaps as a reaction against it, our ancestors were exposed to changing pollen levels from the plants around them. It may have been enough to trigger the allergic potential of our sophisticated immune systems.

This clash of interest a long time ago opened a chink in our armour, and led to the establishment of heightened susceptibility with the potential for the reaction we call hay fever. Today it is acknowledged that hereditary factors predispose sufferers to the complaint.

Enough of pollen. Even an ex-hay fever sufferer is feeling a little uncomfortable! Let us move on to what these little grains actually do to cause discomfort to those of us who are susceptible to them.

A susceptible person will not notice the first crucial contact with pollen. Entering through the nose, the pollen grain is trapped by the hairs in the nostrils and caught on the layer of mucus that coats the flesh. This mucus contains enzymes called lysosomes, which digest trapped particles, breaking them up into tiny fragments. These act on the pollen grain, breaking down that tough horny shell to release the proteins within onto the cells lining the inside of the nose.

The structure of these foreign proteins is registered by the body's immunological system, and if the pollen is judged to be a dangerous invader, the immune system manufactures *antibodies* to render it harmless. This is what the body does if the protein is part of a virus or bacterium.

The antibody then becomes one of a library of specific answers to specific problems. If you are immune to smallpox, it is because your immune system has the appropriate antibody to smallpox on file, ready for use. Small numbers of all the antibodies on file circulate, on patrol, if you like, in the blood and other body fluids.

If the body gets this right and produces antibodies to harmful invaders, we are immune. If, however, it makes a mistake and produces antibodies to harmless invaders such as pollen, then we become sensitised to that pollen. And the next time that pollen is encountered, the immune system will react in a totally inappropriate way.

Because pollen is not a biological invader in the true sense, that is, it does not actively attack body cells or take them over to breed and spread as viruses do, the reaction to it is localised at the site where it was encountered. These are the body cells exposed to the air, and particularly those of the various mucus membranes.

To understand what happens to these cells when we have hay fever, we need to look at the immune system in some detail, to grasp the range, complexity, and wonder of this part of our selves.

The ability of humans — and other animals, for that matter — to resist constant attacks by a wide range of microscopic invaders is something that we are not aware of most of the time. Our immune systems deal with threats ranging from bacteria (germs) and viruses to protozoans (minute single celled animals) and larger parasites, including fungi.

The immune systems work at many levels, and with a variety of mechanisms and options. Their discovery was one of the fascinating stories of medicine. And although their sophistication allows them to deal with the wide range of harmful things listed above, their very complexity must mean that they will occasionally go wrong.

Disease conditions that are believed to be caused by parts of the immune system being over-enthusiastic or running slightly out of control and attacking the body's own cells have been recognised for some time. Common examples are rheumatoid arthritis, ulcerative colitis, and pernicious anaemia.

The working principle which guides the action of the immune system is this: it must decide, at the molecular level, what material is part of the body to which it belongs — 'self', and what is foreign — 'not-self'. The system should then act appropriately, protecting self from not-self.

If the invader contains molecules that give the message, 'not-self, but known', the right immune response will be on file, and produced to deal with the problem. If it is 'not-self, not known', a holding action will be switched on, usually involving interferon, which will protect cells from invasion while the immune system manufactures an appropriate answer.

Another way of dealing with invaders is by chemical warfare. The immune system causes chemical 'mediators' to be released from cells to create a local environment that is hostile to the invader. The temperature of the body may rise to produce an environment that is poorly suited to the invader. And it may be physically attacked and destroyed by specialised cells.

The library of on file answers are the antibodies to specific infectious diseases. These antibodies are themselves protein molecules which take a shape that allows each one to lock onto a specific virus, bacterium, or other invader. They fit precisely together like the pieces of a perfect jigsaw.

Since each type of antibody deals only with the antigen for which it was created, this part of the system is called the *specific immune system*. We acquire some antibodies before birth, and pick up some more in our mother's milk if we are breast fed. Otherwise, we have to develop specific immunity by exposure to disease as we go through life.

The disease organisms, and any other foreign body which causes the immune system to react, are called *antigens*. The reaction is called, logically enough, the antibody-antigen reaction, it is sometimes written as a-a in notes.

47

Antibody protein molecules are called immunoglobulins. Once more, there are a variety of immunoglobulins and they operate in different ways, but those we are concerned with here are the immunoglobulins of class E, normally written as IgE.

Immunoglobulins have to come into contact with the antigens to have any effect. Once they are locked on, there are a variety of ways to take out or neutralise the invader. Some work by weight of numbers; one or two will attach themselves to an antigen and others join up with them to form a criss-cross lattice work. Eventually, the structure becomes so large that it precipitates out of the body fluid as a minute solid which can then be disposed of. In other situations, the fact that an antibody has attached itself seems to be enough to make the antigen give in.

An antibody bound to an antigen may also attach itself to a white blood cell. When this happens, they will be gobbled up together and disposed of. The white cell will also be destroyed, and the resulting outflow of chemicals causes a localised reaction. This attracts other white cells to deal with any other antibody/antigen combinations in the area. When this happens near the surface of the skin, we may be aware of the irritation that results, and notice the debris of the activity as a spot filled with pus.

Our immune systems are in operation all the time, maintaining constant surveillance and keeping our bodies clear of invaders. The body cells, too, are monitored, and those that are incorrect in some way will be removed, for our immune systems are also designed to fight cancer cells.

Usually, we are unaware of this activity, but when our body is fighting an infectious threat we may feel 'one degree under' for a few days while the immune system deals with it. We may find enlarged glands, for example in the neck near the joint of the jaw, for these are mustering points for the white blood cells.

Difficulties arise when the system has to cope with those areas of our bodies which are neither sealed inside, nor totally outside. These interfaces include the orifices that we use to breathe, eat, hear and see through, and they are where the problems arise for hay fever sufferers.

The surfaces of these entry and exit points are lined with a range of specialised cells. These keep them lubricated, clean, and generally act to enable them to fulfil their specialised functions.

One of these duties is to watch out for any hostile organisms that might try to sneak in. This would be bad for the body as a whole, and special cells are there to prevent it.

As part of the watchdog system, our ears, eyes, nose, throat and gut have *mast cells* on their inner surfaces. In their turn,these cells have IgEs attached to them, lying dormant. They will stay there, doing nothing, until the invader that caused the IgE to be created returns.

For the hay fever sufferer, this is the key to the complaint.

Those IgEs are there because of an error. The pollen for which they were created was wrongly identified as a harmful invader. Now it is on file, and IgEs designed to deal with it will always be available, alert, and ready to act whenever it breezes in and makes contact.

A question may spring to the sufferer's mind. Why don't the IgEs simply dispose of the pollen invader, as they would with an infectious invader, without bothering me?

To answer this, and solve last part of the hay fever puzzle, we need to consider the function of those mast cells on which our unwanted IgEs lurk.

What exactly do mast cells do in our bodies? It must be admitted that the details of their biological function remain unclear, and it is therefore the subject of debate. Mast cells are found in many sites of the body in addition to those mentioned earlier. They are present in tissue from the lips right down into our intestines, they are found around the junctions where small veins or arteries join with larger systems, and there is a liberal scattering of them in our skin.

The general medical view of mast cells is that, since they are obviously strategically placed, they must be rapid response sentinels. They guard against possible entry into the body by any foreign body and act to limit the damage caused by injury.

Mast cells are peculiar because they contain relatively large amounts of histamine. This is bound into granules with a chemical called heparin, which prevents blood clotting. Upsetting mast cells causes them to de-granulate, releasing a torrent of chemical mediators into the surrounding intercellular space. This can eventually involve the production of many more chemical mediators. The functions of some of these are known; for example, the kinins are messengers which are involved in producing the

49

sensation of pain. Their role is apparently to make us aware of damage to the cells.

Degranulation will cause local irritation and inflammation. However, if mast cells are provoked to degranulate in many parts of the body at the same time it causes fatal anaphylactic shock.

The mechanism that causes mast cell de-granulation in hay fever sufferers is known. When a pollen grain of the right sort contacts its IgE on the surface of a mast cell and binds to it, it has only to contact another similar IgE on the same cell to cause that cell to degranulate. The bridging effect somehow initiates the reaction in the cell.

In addition to histamine and heparin, with their primary effects, the chemicals released also provoke a wide variety of secondary effects. These will vary depending on the individual concerned and the circumstances at the time. Most people will be aware of the reaction when it happens on some scale involving many cells, and they will produce symptoms of one sort or another.

It is obvious that mast cells have the capacity to regulate a wide range of local events in the body. According to the sentinel view, which follows from the opinion that histamine has a damage control and repair function, they should act in ways which are largely beneficial. But as we all know, this beneficial side of the action can rapidly get out of hand.

In attempts to explain this anomaly, scientists have developed two theories to explain what mast cells are actually supposed to do. As often happens in science, they express opposing views, but both are helpful in understanding some aspects of the hay fever mechanism.

The first theory is that of the degranulators. They hold that mast cells are meant to be activated and to degranulate. This is because their primary function is to cause fatal damage to parasites by flooding them with noxious chemicals when they attempt to invade the body, and that the bridging of the IgEs is the signal for the attack to begin.

If the invader is a parasite, this may be the right thing to do; but when the IgEs have been produced because of a mistake about the true nature of the pollen grain, it may not be helpful at all.

In fact, under these circumstances, firing up the mast cells will be totally inappropriate. Whereas evolution may have tolerated

50

the discomfort of this reaction as part of the price to be paid for bumping off an invader, it is a high price to pay for a case of mistaken identity. However, evolution at all levels is full of such paradoxes.

The second theory, the 'as you were' school, holds that mast cells should not degranulate. Rather, they believe, in just sitting there with their attached IgEs and other immunoglobulins, the mast cells are doing their job.

This theory is clearly more subtle. What are the mast cells doing, then? Two things, apparently.

First, by passing intercellular fluid through the granules in the mast cells, the nature of that fluid is changed. The granules act rather like a filter bed, regulating the chemical messages that are carried in the fluid from cell to cell.

According to the second part of the theory, the IgEs are acting as doormen admitting different protein profiles into a memory store that is actually inside the mast cell. It is speculated that the granules could be acting like the silicon chips in computers, being imprinted with the profiles admitted by the doormen. In this way they give the body a local data base for the recognition of friendly foreign proteins, such as foods, as they pass through the body.

Mast cells burst when the IgE doormen get overloaded and are short circuited.

On reflection, we see no reason why mast cells should not perform both functions. Their normal low-level activity could be to act as memory banks monitoring the passage of various harmless but 'not-self' proteins, while their high level defensive activity could be to react decisively against harmful invaders.

Whatever the scientific truth, it is certain that mast cells have a tremendous capacity to influence all those primary and secondary symptoms familiar to hay fever sufferers.

Histamine is an important product of the high level mast cell reaction. It is released when the cells degranulate or are damaged, and it is also present in small quantities in intercellular fluid. Its normal function seems to be to induce swelling to protect and cushion injuries. If your shoe rubs your foot, histamine causes the affected skin cells to swell. If you continue to walk, the intercellular fluid will accumulate and form a blister, sacrificing the surface skin to protect the flesh beneath.

Similarly, if you cut yourself, the histamine released causes the cells around the wound to swell up to block the site and assist in limiting bleeding. If the damage you suffer is extensive, as in a motor accident, then the excessive amount of histamine released will initiate a shock reaction to immobolise and anaesthetise you to limit self-inflicted secondary damage.

In this role, histamine acts as a finely balanced tool. Under normal circumstances it assists with the control and healing processes involved in local injury. But if histamine is released for the wrong reason, in the wrong place or in the wrong quantity, it causes problems. Then the balance can be hopelessly lost. In massive excess it causes anaphylactic shock; in localised overdose it is responsible for all those hay fever symptoms that victims know so well.

Let us summarise.

The evolution of plants and humans clashed some 20,000 years ago in a way that set up the possibility of hay fever emerging as a disease several thousands of years, and many plant and human generations later.

The scene had been set for this clash by the change of method of pollination forced on plants by the loss of the great tropical forests. The less efficient wind pollination required enormous quantities of pollen to be produced by each flower. Later, humans initiated their own cycle of change by giving up gathering and hunting and settling to agriculture.

From this time onwards, humans have been progressively stressing their environment, the other plants and animals of the planet, and themselves.

It may perhaps seem unfortunate that we evolved such a complex defensive immune system. Like most highly complicated mechanisms, when it works it is wonderful but when it goes wrong it can be an absolute headache.

Allergic disease at all levels, from the subclinical malaise identified by the clinical ecologists, through a variety of recognised illnesses including hay fever, to fatal anaphylaxis, is one of the results of this interaction of factors.

Today the tendency initiated by the chance events of evolution is firmly established. It is also being made more serious each year as more people are being exposed to stresses which allow a widening variety of allergens to breach their adaptive capacity.

For individuals, the network of causes that make them into sufferers looks something like this. They start with an inherited predisposition to react to airborne pollens with hay fever symptoms. This predisposition seems to involve having a significantly higher level of IgE antibodies in their immune systems. At some crucial stage of their personal development which involves a combination of physical and emotional stress and some years of past exposure to pollens, the system suffers overload. The familiar malfunction is initiated.

We all have very similar immune systems. The potential for failing to adapt to environmental stress and thus beginning to malfunction exists within us all.

Everyone has a last straw.

For those predisposed to hay fever, the conditions under which most people live in western industrialised nations, with the effluent of industrial processes and a way of life which annually increases the stress loading on individuals, it is little wonder that more people every year reach their limit.

The point where increasing susceptibility is matched by the appearance of large quantities of a particular pollen, with a protein coat which the IgEs decide is just too much, is reached. The first sneeze or buzzing in the ears heralds hay fever triggered in yet another individual.

Once the IgEs and their associated mast cells have been fired up by a pollen trigger, things can only get worse. The sensitisation which happened quietly some time before has produced militant IgE antibodies which are now reacting. The resultant outpouring of histamine produces the uncomfortable symptoms.

Once the membranes involved are in turmoil, any similar pollen or indeed other allergen will add to the problem. A vicious circle is established. Once mast cells have been triggered, degranulated, and caused the surrounding tissues to become sensitive, they will not only react more quickly next time they encounter that particular pollen, but will tend to react to a wider range of pollens.

Triggered pollen sensitivity leads to increased pollen sensitivity. Some limit will be reached; it is rare for people to become sensitive to all pollens. The suffering will also reach a limit, but while the inflamed tissues are exposed to pollen they will go on reacting, becoming red and sore. Exposure does not allow

53

time for the swelling to subside and the tissues to heal.

As far as the mast cells are concerned, they are doing a good job. They are preventing harmful foreign bodies entering the body by trapping them on the mucous membranes, which they see as being under continual attack.

Part of the local defence strategy involves bathing the tissues in fluids. Usually these take the form of excessive amounts of the fluids naturally produced at the particular site. Ears get waxier, eyes wetter, and more mucous is produced in the nose and throat.

Eventually the stability of the battlefield is reached. You may wish to class yourself as a non-combatant, but as far as your immune system is concerned, it, together with its various allies, is holding the enemy at bay. They are protecting you from an infection.

If the primary cause of a particular individual's suffering is genetic, then perhaps little can be done about it. But the increase in the number of hay fever cases each year cannot be blamed entirely on inheritance of the condition. We must look elsewhere for significant contributions to the increasing susceptibility to allergic reactions experienced among the population as a whole.

In our general look at hay fever in Chapter One, we mentioned that some people blamed the growing use of petrol engines in motor vehicles for the increase in the disease. This was a move in the right direction, but the focus was too narrow. Behind the growing use of petrol and motor vehicles is the parallel growth of the petro-chemical industry itself.

This industry hardly existed at the beginning of the twentieth century. Now it consists of some of the biggest, richest and most powerful multi-national businesses in the world. Their rise to such spectacular pre-eminence is not only because we all want to drive cars and need petrol. It is because they are in the business of actually inventing synthetic materials which would not normally exist in nature.

Industrial chemists found that they could join molecules together in an almost infinite number of ways to produce entirely new substances. These include all the plastics, many drugs, and artificial fibres, as well as many other things that we take for granted. At the time of invention what a substance turns out to be is frequently a matter of chance. It might be a new drug, a paint solvent, food additive, lubricant, shoe polish, fertiliser or a miracle hair restorer. Because of the unpredictable nature of the products, the process is known as 'molecular roulette'.

The number of these substances available is staggering. There are over four million on the computer register of the American Chemical Abstract Service, and of these around 35,000 are in everday use in most parts of the world. In this context 'everyday use' means although widespread, they may have been in existence for no more than perhaps two or three decades.

The problem for possible hay fever sufferers is that exposure to *any* substance that our immune system can regard with suspicion can move them progressively nearer to the triggering point.

Although all these substances will be passed as safe, that is really meaningless in this context. What, after all, could be much safer than a pint of milk? The answer is nothing — as long as *you* are not allergic to it!

From time to time specific substances pop up which are unquestionably hazardous. Thalidomide is an example from the drug industry, now known all over the world. Additionally there are many which are controversial, such as the herbicide 2–4–5T. This chemical was widely used in forestry before it was suggested that it induced spontaneous abortion, or led to the birth of deformed children. Some countries banned it, others did not. From those substances which turn out to be obviously dangerous the scale of risk rapidly slides into grey areas of doubt.

It must be acknowledged that few of us could live the lives that we do without the myriad products of the chemical industry. We may have to accept that a growing burden of ill-health among the population at large is an unavoidable part of the price for the products and lifestyle we wish to enjoy.

Does this mean that we must simply accept hay fever, or muddle through it as best we can?

Of course not!

But it does mean we have a three-cornered fight on our hands. Firstly there is the problem of our individual susceptibility, and there may be quite a lot we can do about that, despite its apparently immutable genetic base.

Next there is the problem of the frighteningly large number of possible background and environmental allergens, which help to raise and maintain our susceptibility.

Their activity in this respect may be complicated by the subtle addictive effect that they have on us. It is not often realised that part of the adaptive process to the stress these substances impose can involve becoming addicted to them. The stress produces a little rush of adrenalin, which gives us a pleasant lift. After a while we welcome the offender and suffer withdrawal symptoms if it is removed.

This 'acceptable' pollution is a complex question. It demands long term answers based on a true appreciation of the problem it presents.

What is certain is that there is little point in seeking a cure or relief from the obvious effects of a particular pollen, if the wider circumstances that made us its victim remain unchanged.

The problem is only likely to return, perhaps in a different form, because the causal stress will still be affecting us.

Finally we come to the plants and their pollen.

Here we must think about ecology in its widest sense. While there are many sources of concerned comment about the plight of this species of animal, or that particular part of the global habitat — all of which is to be welcomed — few commentators point to the underlying mechanism which is causing the problems.

Every species of life has its own peculiar *morphology* — literally, the shape of the species as a whole. It is known that if the number of animals of any species falls below a certain figure, they will die out. The species needs a certain level of population for it to be viable.

This is because when numbers drop below the viable level the morphology of the species has been distorted too much for it to recover. The problem is seen most obviously with the difficulty experienced in getting some animals to breed in isolated pairs in zoos. In some way the pair is not sufficiently complete to continue.

Scientists are beginning to explore the proposition that *all* members of the same species are in some way connected to all other members.

In the case of humans this connectedness, the strength of our shared morphology, is being measured in terms of changed learning rates. Rupert Sheldrake, who has been developing this theory, has been carrying out research into mass recognition of

56

ambiguous images. You may have seen an abstract picture that was shown on TV in late 1983 as part of an international experiment. The proposition seems to be supported, that we are influenced by other members of our species in ways that we are learning to measure but cannot yet fully explain.

If the assertion that every species has a similar shared morphology is accepted, then the antagonistic quality of a growing number of plant pollens, and their sheer quantity, may reflect the collective desperation of increasing numbers of plant species. What we are doing to the environment we share with them could be provoking them to react.

Inflicting hay fever may be one of the few ways they can fight back.

4 Dealing with hay fever

Our examination of the cause of hay fever within the body might seem to imply that dealing with the condition should be simple. We just need to get in among the pollens, mast cells, and IgEs, and assert some control over their interaction.

A moment of reflection will reveal that it cannot be that simple. Such control may contribute part of the picture for some individuals, but it is unlikely to provide the whole answer for anyone. It is far too simplistic an approach for the nature of the disease and the interacting pressures that cause it.

Our approach needs to be both general, involving a consideration of the large background factors concerned in the condition, and at the same time particular. Sufferers need to locate by experience as many as possible of the things that contribute to their own hay fever reaction, and eliminate or treat them.

As with many diseases that are produced or made worse by conditions in modern society, the approach to treatment has to be two-pronged. If it simply stops at curing the immediate symptoms, the potential for ill-health caused by the same pressures remains, and will tend to emerge in another, perhaps worse, form. Treating any disease without attacking its cause is at best an unsatisfactory stop-gap, and should not be seen as anything more.

We shall deal with the possibilities of cures in the accepted sense in some detail in later chapters. However, there is no single safe and generally effective method known to medicine that will work for all hay fever victims, whatever the approach taken.

The problem with medical treatment is that it involves interfering with the actions of body systems that we need in order to resist infection and remain healthy. The mast cells and their attached immunoglobulins play a role that is far too important to ignore. Although we may resent their propensity to over-react, we should not survive if they ceased to react at all. So a breakthrough in biochemical manipulation that will produce a totally satisfactory solution to the hay fever problem seems extremely unlikely.

No responsible allergist would propose that any hay fever sufferer should rely on medicine alone without doing everything possible to reduce the severity of the complaint first.

The ideal answer, of course, would be to persuade the mast cells to be more selective in their choice of IgEs. But until we know how to influence them in this way, the best we can do is reduce their general tendency to over react.

Because hay fever is a comparatively modern complaint, it lacks the wealth of traditional remedies that such conditions usually collect. With the growth in numbers of sufferers, some personal methods of symptomatic relief have evolved; and almost every season there is a newspaper or TV feature about the latest one.

While some of these may be amusing or spectacular, very few seem to stand the test of time and none has come into widespread use. However they involve little risk and may have some value. If they work for you, they work, and are therefore worth considering.

Many people find that irritation of the eyes, which is particularly unpleasant on bright, clear, sunny days, can be alleviated by wearing sunglasses. Whether this is because the glare effect on sensitised tissues is reduced, or because the glasses prevent some pollen from reaching the eyes by acting as windscreens, is not clear. It could be a combination of both. The problem with this approach used to be that when you came indoors, you had to take your sunglasses off to see where you were going. Modern light-reactive glasses have removed this minor drawback.

For those whose problem is the sore, sometimes raw, throat and the coughing that can accompany hay fever, warm honey drinks can be helpful. Some people maintain that this is because of the bee-pollen-honey relationship. Beneficial actions are attributed to the effects of honey on the mast cells, treating like with like much as homoeopathy does.

It seems more likely that the drink washes away the chemical debris of mast cell degranulation, giving the throat some rest before it all starts up again. They may possibly assist in providing an insulating layer between the cells and the air passing over them, and the warmth can be soothing. But for those with a weight or diet problem, honey drinks are not a good idea.

Sucking sweets, including cough sweets, has similar effects and similar drawbacks. Liquorice can be helpful; its derivatives are actually used in medicine to treat stomach ulcers, in which histamine is also implicated, but it is not known how it works. In high doses, liquorice can produce serious side-effects including high blood pressure, heart irregularities and muscles weakness. Don't overdo it — it is a potent drug. Certainly, strong liquorice will promote salivation, and this in itself is helpful. For those who dislike liquorice or would rather not actually eat anything, an alternative is to suck a nut. This will be enough to stimulate the flow of saliva.

Cough syrups offer a compromise between medicines and sweets. Many brands are available over the counter in chemists' shops, and some will provide marginal relief for hay fever symptoms. Many contain an antihistamine as one of the main active ingredients. The syrup content is there less for therapeutic reasons than to make the potion more attractive.

The use of sweet syrups as drug carriers can cause problems for those who find it difficult to resist sweet things, particularly when they are offered the excuse that it is 'medicinal'. The danger is of unintended overdose. Since a hay fever sufferer is likely to be taking antihistamines in another form, this could cause more of the all too familiar drowsiness and unwanted sleep problems.

Other 'cold cures', such as nasal decongestants, are also used for self-medication by sufferers for whom a runny nose is a particular problem. Their use demands particular care, and they are discussed fully in the next chapter.

At the other extreme of self-medication, the once ubiquitous vaseline petroleum jelly has some advocates. It is claimed that a light smear of jelly around the nostrils can reduce the symptoms. It is conceivable that for some people a layer of grease strategically placed could act as a sort of pollen trap.

If all else fails the hay fever sufferer can hide. When things are particularly bad, perhaps because of a short sharp reaction to particularly high levels of pollen, the only thing to do is retire. The tranquillity of a cool dark room can be enhanced with a damp towel over the face or bathing with cold water.

These do-it-yourself methods of suppressing hay fever symptoms can work for some people under some conditions. While they may all be worth remembering and trying, there is little documented evidence of their effectiveness to guide sufferers. They are most likely to be useful to those who have a low level of susceptibility and whose symptoms respond fairly easily.

For most sufferers, something more is needed. It remains true that, once hay fever has them in its grip, they will try almost anything, no matter how limited or ludicrous, to gain relief. These people will have to take more far-reaching action to control their hay fever.

What can we do to deal with some of the broader influences on hay fever?

As with all disease, the better your general health, the less you are likely to suffer. The frequently ignored rules for a healthy life apply to hay fever sufferers as much as to anyone else: unfortunately they are also ignored by sufferers just as much. It is perhaps only natural for them to breathe a long sigh of relief at the end of the pollen season, feeling so much better, relatively, that they will put everything to do with the problem firmly out of their minds. Until next year, of course.

The wise course of action is to take action against hay fever *before* the season starts.

Staying healthy means taking positive action. The way we are encouraged to live in modern society, particularly in cities, is not at all healthy. We live in bodies designed for action but cars, escalators, lifts, and all the provisions of public transport, rob us of the ability even to walk any distance, let alone run. Our muscles, including our hearts, deteriorate through under-use. We suffer premature metabolic senility, growing old before our time.

Leisure and luxury, which generally mean doing nothing in the easiest possible way, are sold as desirable ways of living. The truth is that ease and convenience are often against our best interests. To be healthy, we should live active and fulfilling lives.

The British as a whole are well known for their determined hatred of exercise. Perhaps this is because the word conjures up unpleasant memories of cold knees and ridicule at school. Whatever the reason, there is no doubt that our attitude to fitness leads us to suffer from all sorts of diseases that could easily be avoided.

We have been encouraged by thirty-five years of National Health Services to believe that we can abuse or ignore our health in any way we choose. We just take the results along to the doctor or hospital to have it all put back together again.

The ineffectiveness of this approach is all too obvious from the statistics. A recent survey of the British people showed that only 23% of men and 15% of women could report no illness whatever in the fortnight before they were interviewed. Chronic ill-health is more common than good health.

Fortunately many people are becoming realistic about the limits of medical care, and concluding that it is far better to stay healthy.

We need to change our *attitude* to ourselves, taking pride and pleasure in our bodies and abilities. Life is a once only experience and we get much more out of it when we put in a little more.

Positive health action for hay fever sufferers should include minimising exposure to artificial substances that increase allergic potential. While it is obviously impossible to avoid exposure to the outside world, a lot can be achieved in the immediate personal and home environment.

What you eat might be a good place to start. Although many hay fever sufferers may not be allergic to foods, any allergies they do have will contribute to their allergic load. Hay fever sufferers may be sensitive to dairy foods, wheat, eggs, beef and pork, in that order. In Ireland, some specialists have successfully treated sufferers by eliminating all dairy products from their diet. It may be well worthwhile exploring the possibility that you have an allergic reaction to a common food that launches you into hay fever each year.

Even if this does not provide dramatic relief, there is little point in suffering a food allergy since they are avoidable. There are numerous books available which deal specifically with food allergies. If you suspect that a sub-clinical condition, or even a major illness, may be connected with the food you eat, it is well worth taking the time and trouble to investigate the possibility.

The discussion of food and health is a contentious one, even if the question of specific allergies is excluded. But some basic rules have emerged through the welter of conflicting claims.

The British diet contains too much sugar and too much salt.

You are probably aware of this, and may try to cut back on your consumption, but it isn't easy unless you decide to avoid processed food. Nearly all processed foods have sugar and salt added when they are prepared and refined. This is good for sales because we are all programmed to seek these substances. They are rare in nature and our ancestors needed to get them when they could, but in civilisation they are over-abundant and their inclusion encourages *addiction* to foods which contain excessive amounts.

The bad health that results ranges from heart attacks to nervous and behavioural disorders. We were not designed to cope with the amounts of these substances that our modern diet contains.

The harmful effects of excessive sugar and salt are intensified by another widespread eating error, the over consumption of animal fat. Once again, these are substances that we would meet only rarely in nature. Wild animals, roaming over large areas, do not run to fat.

While not wishing to go deeply into these questions in this book, we would ask you to accept this. The overwhelming consensus among people with no commercial interest, is that minimising consumption of all these substances will improve your survival chances and general health.

The guiding rule is this. The more highly processed, prepared, and packaged the food is, the more harmful junk it is likely to contain. In addition to sugar and salt, the additives include artificial colourings, preservatives, stabilisers, and flavourings. Fast food tops the junk table, and in our opinion should be totally avoided.

Healthy eating is rooted in common sense. It is easy to get food that has been subjected to the minimum of interference. Just ignore the blandishments of the bright lights and the advertisements that offer a new way of life/romance/leisure or instant transfer to an exotic part of the world with every packet. Aim for *real* food, as fresh as possible, and a diet that includes a wide range of basic fruit and vegetables.

In the immediate personal environment, the most obvious area for attack to improve your health is that of domestic cleaning.

No, this is not a plea for more vigilance in washing, dusting, scouring and polishing. Rather the reverse, for with the exception of vacuum cleaning, few of these domestic activities actually benefit the hay fever sufferer. In fact, they may exacerbate the condition.

A look at the vast range of powders, liquids, pastes, polishes, sprays, foams, and creams available to the conscientious housewife in every grocery and supermarket gives a clue to the size of the problem.

For us, just walking through one of these 'allergen alleys' is enough to provoke a sneeze or two. If the advertisers are to be believed, missing the advantages claimed for some of these products can be tantamount to a severe dereliction of wifely duty. The possible consequences border on the death of the entire family, though whether from shame or from unspecified but deadly disease, is not clear.

This over-obsession with a germ-free environment stems from the discovery of the importance of a few microbes in certain disease processes. Louis Pasteur, the French chemist who gave us pasteurised milk, discovered the importance of the micro-sphere to a variety of life processes.

The Victorians believed that hygiene was very important in defeating disease, and indeed the magnificent water and sewage works they built did play a crucial role in improving the life expectancy of the population. However, our attitudes to hygiene today, bordering as they do on the obsessive, indicate that there has been something of an over-reaction.

The modern view is more realistic. If we were actually to 'kill all known germs — *dead*', we should follow soon afterwards. We depend on the operation of microbes for the essential life processes on this planet. Their activity sustains all other life forms.

While dirt does promote biological activity, and can indeed harbour disease, we do not need to be constantly scrubbing, mopping, spraying, polishing and disinfecting our environment to remain healthy.

We may object to dirt on aesthetic grounds. In most circumstances it is much more likely to offend our eyes than harm our bodies. In fact, the amount of chemical pollution we deposit in our immediate environment keeping it 'clean' is likely to be a major contributor to the subclinical disease experienced by many housewives. It is also likely to be an added factor in precipitating allergic reactions among hay fever sufferers.

This is not a suggestion that you become slovenly. Nor is it a moralistic plea that you subject yourself to the drudgery of grandmother's day — though many modern housewives might be interested to know that they spend just as many hours on housework, despite modern conveniences, as their grandmothers did.

Once more, common sense is the best answer. The number of things we really need to keep clean and polished in our homes are very few. Try cutting back on the number of cleaning products you use; not only will it save money, but it could make a surprising difference to the way you feel. The frequency of those apparently random headaches may be a good indicator. In Norway, people who are being considered for hyposensitisation treatment for allergies, including hay fever, are first given a booklet listing a range of household products that must be removed from the home environment before treatment is allowed to begin. This list includes a variety of detergent washing powders, some paints, fabrics, floor coverings, furniture fillings, and other products which cause allergy in some people.

Apart from vacuuming, most cleaning can be managed with a little plain soap and water, or just a damp cloth. Washing may need detergents, but remember that liquids will put less into the air you breathe than powders. The results may not always be so spectacular, but your health will benefit.

The general rule should be to go for the simplest and most direct method. Don't use noxious 'air fresheners' — use the real thing — fresh air!

Which brings us to the problem of tobacco smoke.

Smoking is the single largest cause of ill health under individual control.

In the United States, three independent Commissions, reporting to three different Presidents, each strongly recommended that tobacco should be banned outright because of its disastrous effects on health. Not only is smoking clearly associated with lung cancer and heart disease, but it also causes other serious problems. These range from blood vessel disease which requires progressive surgical pruning of the victims' limbs, to a greatly increased susceptibility to all kinds of infectious disease and many cancers.

Since tobacco smoke directly irritates the respiratory system, the nose and throat as well as the lungs, it is particularly implicated in respiratory disease. Smokers are much more likely to develop any infection or malfunction in the respiratory system, from colds and sore throats to bronchitis and emphysema.

Nicotine is a very dangerous and highly addictive drug. Despite the impression given by the popular media, the effects of heroin on the health of the nation are minimal in comparison to those of tobacco. Yet despite this, governments have felt unable to act in the face of a powerful tobacco industry lobby and the political pressure of millions of addicts.

In Britain the conflict of interest expresses itself as confusion. After three decades in which the number of smokers has slowly but steadily declined, smoking is now a minority habit. Nevertheless it is difficult to find public places that are not heavily polluted. And the remaining smokers still assume an inalienable right to pollute our bodies secondhand, while they poison their own at first hand.

Some hay fever sufferers have a peculiar love-hate relationship with smoking. For them, the very thought of a cigarette in the pollen season is like the threat of death, but once the season is over they will smoke quite happily. From personal experience we know that if you don't start up again in the autumn, the hay fever symptoms are not so bad the following spring.

To carry on smoking through the hay fever season will inevitably worsen the symptoms. Tobacco smoke irritates the inflamed membranes even more. Those smokers who are so addicted that they will knowingly subject themselves to this might ask themselves whether the short-term misery of giving up for good would really be worse than this annual torture.

The best advice for everyone, but especially for hay fever sufferers, is not to smoke, and to avoid those places where passive smoking is forced on you.

Now in case you are beginning to think that all of the foregoing advice is some sort of plea for a return to natural living, perhaps conjuring up pictures of weaving, living 'the good life', brewing your own beer, and surviving on a smallholding producing lots of earthy vegetables, let us just say this. For all our illusions of a civilisation insulated by a dominant technology, we cannot divorce ourselves from that nature of which we are a part. Every step we take away from a natural life has a price which we pay in ill-health and premature death.

While it would obviously be impossible for us all to depart into some rural idyll, even if we wanted to, the underlying reality of our nature cannot be ignored. The perspective we should grasp is that practically all disease apart from that we were born with is the result of the breakdown of one of the systems of the body or mind. There are enough things which can cause such breakdowns without us going out of our way to help. In fact, we should be pushing as hard as we can in the opposite direction.

Why do we need to take account of all these things when dealing with hay fever? The basic rationale is quite simple: the more we can do to counter the *causes* of disease, the better.

Of the nine million plus British hay fever victims, many could have their condition considerably improved by living in a better human environment. Perhaps many need never have become susceptible in the first place. Turning off the taps that contribute to the disease stream is far better than waiting until millions are ill, then vainly trying to find cures.

If turning off the immediate disease taps seems too big a task, what about turning off the individual ones? What about the possibility of *avoiding* the pollens that trigger the reaction?

In the summer of 1982, some people were trying this approach. You may have seen pictures of them on TV or in the papers, carefree in their goldfish bowl space helmets with associated air filter and pump backpack connected by a flexible pipe.

Now while we would not wish to disparage any measure which would bring relief to hay fever sufferers, the essence of the condition for most people is that it is life-limiting. If your life could be made less limited by becoming an alien on your own planet, with all the problems of eating, drinking, and inter-human contact that this implies, then give it a try. Perhaps you will benefit. One reporter who tested them for social acceptability was surprised at how few people laughed, but was disturbed by the 'greenhouse effect' of the helmet which made it almost too hot to wear outside on sunny days.

Carrying your own mini-controlled environment around on your head would be totally unnecessary if you could avoid venturing outside, and instead adapt your indoor environment to your needs. This involves pollen-proofing your house. Effectively, shutting all windows and doors, stopping draughts, and blocking chimneys. Realistically, one room could be treated fully and the remainder of the house regarded as a series of ante-chambers.

Fortunately, because pollen levels show regular variations over the course of the day, it is possible to air the house at carefully regulated times when the outside pollen level is at its lowest. To do this effectively, you will need to discover which pollens cause you to react, and monitor their effects carefully over a long enough period to be able to judge when you can risk opening windows. For example, if you are allergic to grass pollens, you should be reasonably safe in the early hours of the morning.

Even without taking such great care, pollen levels inside buildings can generally remain very much lower than those outside if the windows are kept shut, and air movement reduced to a minimum. Clearly, the effectiveness of this strategy will vary with the size and layout of the building.

Under favourable circumstances, the effect of staying indoors can be very marked. For example, the pollen count on the roof of a high building in Cardiff was found to be, on average, fifty times higher than that in a closed room nearby.

Having pollen-proofed the house as far as possible, the hay fever sufferer can then deal with the pollen that remains in the circulating air. House plant lovers will be relieved to know that they need not get rid of traditional indoor plants; these do not produce airborne pollens.

Air conditioning has been shown to reduce pollen to 2.5% of the outdoor level, and some filters can offer similar benefits. However, the efficiency of the device inevitably varies with its design. Air conditioning is a term that is used to cover a multitude of activities, ranging from simply heating or cooling the air, to filtering, changing its humidity, and altering its temperature. Obviously, the more you do, the more expensive it is.

Air purifiers, sold to remove smells, take two forms. The chemical devices that come in blocks, with wicks and the like, have no effect on pollen levels and should be avoided because they add more chemicals to the environment.

There are also electrostatic devices which claim to be capable of removing pollen and tobacco smoke from the air. According to work published in academic literature a decade ago, they have no measurable effect; but we acknowledge that progress has probably been made since that time. Although the manufacturers maintain that they do reduce pollen levels, they have not been able to provide us with any data to support these claims. We would expect that they could remove some pollen from the air, but that the effect would be localised and limited.

Probably the most effective method of clearing pollen from the air is to use an ionizer. These can reduce the pollen level by causing particles to be precipitated out of the air so that they can be removed from surfaces with damp cloths or by vacuum cleaning.

Basically, ionizers send out a stream of negatively charged air. The negative ions surround particles — including pollen, bacteria, smoke, and dust — and gives them a tiny negative electrical charge. They are then attracted to any positively charged surface, of which there are many in most houses. The particles will turn up particularly on polished surfaces, TV screens, and anything made of synthetic fibre.

Of course, this means that an ionizer will tend to make polished furniture dusty, unless you get a de-luxe model that filters the air as well.

According to research sponsored by ionizer manufacturers Medion, and carried out by Dr Leslie Hawkins of Surrey University, 23% of a sample of a thousand Medion users bought their ionizers in the hope of achieving relief from hay fever. 71% reported definite benefit; 19% felt the ionizer had produced no change, while 8% didn't know whether it had made any difference. Only 2% considered that their symptoms were worse. A similar proportion of users who suffered from other respiratory problems reported benefits.

We tried an ionizer in the Spring of 1984 (see postscript). We noticed no clear benefit, but our experience cannot be considered conclusive. Ionizers were originally promoted because they make the air more refreshing and aid alertness. They have now been shown to produce profound changes in body chemistry. People suffering from allergic conditions can feel better within minutes of using an ionizer, probably because it can reduce blood histamine and serotonin levels.

The manufacturers recommend that hay fever sufferers should

ideally use an ionizer every night in the bedroom from February onwards in order to prevent symptoms beginning in May. Then, during the summer, they can be used as desired to clear the pollen from the air.

Most ionizers are quite small devices. Some are designed to be used in cars; others, intended for office or factory use, can produce a stream of ions covering quite large areas. It is important, however, to choose a model produced by a reputable manufacturer, because poorly designed devices have been found to produce ozone (which can be toxic) and very few negative ions.

There are companies that offer a money-back guarantee on their ionizers, so it is possible to use one for a trial period to find out if it is the answer for you.

Alternatively, if you are in London, you could try spending some time in the Underground. It is said that the electrical system produces such a high concentration of negative ions that it has markedly beneficial effects on the health of employees.

Strategies for avoiding pollens could be taken to extremes. The thought of living in an environment with permanently clean and sterile air may appeal, particularly during the hay fever season. But pursuit of this ideal, which has its seeds in large air conditioned buildings and enclosed multi-level shopping centres, parallels the aim of killing all known germs: it assumes that we can divorce ourselves from the biosphere. This is an illusion which denies our basic nature. It usually brings more problems than answers. Despite its superficial attractions and technical feasibility, it is not a route that we should consider.

Understanding the workings of the biosphere can offer more benefits than attempting to dominate it. For hay fever sufferers, this includes finding out precisely how the levels of the particular pollens to which they are allergic fluctuate during the course of the day.

Most plants behave in a very predictable manner, scattering their pollen at the same time every day. The rise and fall of pollen levels from hour to hour can produce pollen counts which vary a hundredfold within the course of twenty four hours. Each species has a peak time.

Unfortunately, this information is not available from tables from which you can read off the safe times, because it varies from place to place. For example, Berkshire stinging nettles have their pollen peak between noon and 1pm, while the stinging nettles around Cardiff peak at 5pm.

Grass pollens principally peak in the early afternoon, though some species have a double maximum, in the late morning and mid-afternoon. The local geography of the London basin produces a relatively late grass pollen peak. Usually it comes at around 7pm. Some weeds, including plantain, peak in the morning. Birch, pine, oak, and ash have morning peaks, while elm (and sometimes oak and ash too) produces its maximum pollen output around midnight.

Weather conditions also have marked effects on pollen levels. Rain can cause some flowers to close and withhold their pollen, and fine rain will scrub the pollen out of the air, cleansing it to allow hay fever sufferers to emerge safely. But beware! The scattered, heavy drops of a thunder shower may remove very little of the pollen from the air.

Some people may find it worthwhile moving house in order to avoid the particular pollen to which they are especially sensitive. High concentrations of pollens can be very local occurrences indeed; a valley will have different plants in it from those that grow on higher land on either side, for example, and local weather conditions may be such that the pollens from the high ground are rarely blown down to the low ground, while valley floor pollens are present in profusion.

Dr John Mullins, of the asthma research unit at Sully Hospital in South Wales, wrote in a letter to us: 'Places a few yards apart may experience different pollen concentrations, as pollen tends to travel in clouds and these clouds are greatly influenced by local atmospheric conditions, eg thermals, eddies, etc, and a study of airborne allergens takes one more and more into the realms of the meterologist.

'There will also be the influence of local sources of allergens. An example which comes to mind is of a Cardiff girl complaining of symptoms during the 'tree' season which shared a good correlation with Hazel pollen, although from our counts in the centre of Cardiff there did not appear to be sufficient pollen to cause her any bother. An investigation of her home circumstances showed that the estate where she lived was built over an area of mature woodland from which stands of trees including mature Hazel were left. She also had hay fever and 50 yards from her house

71

Timothy grass was growing to waist height over an area of rough land. She solved her problems herself by moving back to mother.'

The personal strategy of avoidance can be approached in any of the ways described above, and it will be effective to some degree. But it remains true that any of them will be more effective if action is also taken to reduce your susceptibility threshold.

Increasing your resistance to reaction, by reducing the loading on your system, will make the pollen less of a problem.

Earlier in this chapter we discussed the effects of pollution in the immediate environment in increasing susceptibility to reaction. What was said of the personal environment is equally true of the wider environment which we all share.

Pollen is the last straw for a system which has been stressed by pollution to the point where its susceptibility is matched by an appropriate allergen trigger.

Does it make sense to remove the last straw, and leave the rest of the load?

In 1968, an Italian industrialist gathered a group of world experts at a meeting in Rome. He wanted them to explore the present and future wider predicaments of humanity. The organisation he formed became known as the Club of Rome, and it has used all the power of modern computing science to build predictive models of things that influence our lives. They have developed pictures of global systems of economics, politics, and the natural and social forces at work.

In their ongoing studies throughout the 1970s, the Club of Rome have consistently indicated two sources of disaster for humanity. The first is the unchecked growth of human population, with its demands on resources, which causes the increasing pressure on all other life forms described in the previous chapter. It is customary for us to assume that this is a problem for 'others', usually in Asia and Africa. This is an illusion. Any country that cannot feed itself is overpopulated. In Britain, despite the various EEC mountains, we have to import roughly half our food.

The second disaster area is linked to the first. If more and more people demand more and more manufactured goods and services, the consumption of energy and materials will cause us to die, poisoned by the massive amounts of pollution these processes produce. Hay fever sufferers are a tip of this iceberg of growing environmental ill health.

Clinical ecologists have recently started to explore the disease burden placed on society by things we have generally assumed to be good. These range from food additives through artificial fibres to gas fires. Yet it remains true that there is no accurate measurement of the sickness caused by acknowledged pollution.

However, the National Academy of Sciences in the United States has estimated that 1% of deaths in urban areas of America can be directly attributed to dirty air.

The damage done in recent decades to the Taj Mahal, the Acropolis, and to priceless monuments all over the world by pollution in the air is all too obvious. Our bodies are far less resilient than stone.

Human activities have created a situation in which we all suffer some degree of environmental disease. It may be nothing more than increased susceptibility to colds, or it can be more insidious long term problems like cancer.

Our attitudes must change. We cannot be healthy in an environment which we continually degrade. We must stop treating the land, the sea, and particularly the air, as a giant dustbin. Nobody wants to live in a dustbin, yet we all contribute to the processes that are turning our world into one.

In the long term, a clean, chemical-free environment may be the only answer, not only for hay fever sufferers, but for many other people with related diseases. Hay fever was a little known disease at the beginning of the industrial revolution. In less than two hundred years it has grown to affect countless millions of people. The number of sufferers cannot be accounted for by the spread of unfavourable genes among the population.

Whether the rise of the disease is due to the direct effect of industrial pollution on humans, as seems most probable, or whether it is because of the effect of pollution and environmental changes on plants, or possibly a combination of both, it is a fact that hay fever has grown with the increase in industrial activity and pollution.

The long term options appear to be these. Either we rationalise our demands on our planet and its resources and reduce the pressure of our species' morphology on that of other life forms, or we continue at an accelerating rate to destroy our environment and a progressively larger proportion of the human race with it.

Failure to modify our effect on the planet conjures up a nightmare vision that hay fever sufferers may have an insight into: living in an incapacitated way for longer periods of a lifespan that is being steadily shortened by forces out of control.

Under these circumstances, the rich and privileged will seek survival in medical ghettos, where the artificiality of the life reflects the artificiality of the devastated world outside.

5   Does medicine have an answer?

The medical approach to any health problem is fairly consistent. Generally, some form of drug therapy is sought which will relieve the symptoms of the disorder.

Although we may think in terms of 'curative' and 'preventative' medicine, the reality of treatment today is palliative. Cures are actually very rare indeed. Even antibiotics, which can specifically attack the bacteria which produce infection, will not actually *cure* the illness for which they are taken unless the body's defences are capable of seeking out and eliminating the elusive micro-organisms that remain after the majority have been killed by the drug.

In other words, even our most effective forms of medical treatment depend on the integrity of the healing systems in our own bodies. It is when these, the immune systems, are not functioning properly that the most difficult problems with treatment arise, for scientists do not understand enough about how they work and what factors affect them to be able to predict how to deal with malfunctions.

Although the activity of the immune systems can be suppressed with drugs, such sledge-hammer treatment is very hazardous. Nevertheless it is used under some circumstances — including, regrettably, therapy for severe hay fever.

A prevalent myth in our culture is that drug treatment has saved millions of lives and that we live longer than did our forefathers primarily because of the marvellous achievements of modern medicine. But when the evidence is examined with care and a critical eye, the opposite conclusion appears more probable.

We are convinced that drug treatment today does more harm than good. The number of lives lost through unnecessary and irrational use of potent medicines outnumbers those saved by the appropriate use of these products. In our book, *Cured to Death*, we explain the reasons for this view.

For all that, we would not dismiss western medicine and its application of drug therapy as useless. Far from it. These sophisticated products have real value. But they also have dangers. When they are used, it should be with *full knowledge* of their possible hazards, and only when safer alternatives have been fully explored.

It does not make sense to use drugs as the first approach to therapy.

The fundamental problem with drug therapy is this: for a drug to have an effect it must also have hazards. There is no such thing as a totally safe drug. Every drug has a range of effects on the body. It does not only affect the symptoms for which it is taken.

If you take a pill to deal with hay fever, that drug will be taken up by the tissues involved in producing the symptoms. But it will also spread throughout the body, affecting all the systems that have similar biochemical characteristics. It may, in addition, have some effects on systems which seem entirely unrelated to the organs it is intended to affect. For example, drugs are normally broken down into simpler chemicals in the liver, and eliminated from the body via the kidneys. Many drugs can affect these organs when they accumulate in them, and some can cause serious damage. Opren is perhaps the best-known recent example; prescribed to relieve arthritis, it caused death through liver damage.

Apart from whatever therapeutic effects it may have, each drug will also have *side-effects* and be capable of inducing *adverse reactions* — unintended and unpleasant effects of treatment. Some of these effects are predictable. These are the common, well-recognised side-effects of the drug. However, many adverse reactions are referred to as 'idiosyncratic': they are characteristically unpredictable, unexpected, and uncommon. The dividing line between an unwanted side-effect and an adverse drug reaction is very hazy.

The totally safe drug is a myth. Benefits are always balanced by some risk, and no amount of testing or consumer pressure can produce total drug safety because this balance is inherent in the way drugs act. The least dangerous are those which are applied to very limited areas of the body, and which do not go through any biochemical changes, but are simply excreted.

One of these extremely rare products, sodium cromoglycate, is actually used for hay fever; it is described later in this chapter.

Regrettably, neither the public nor the medical profession seem to be sufficiently aware of the significance of these issues. The persuasive power of the drug manufacturers — who naturally wish to sell their products in massive quantities — combine with the assumptions of our culture to produce a situation where drugs are prescribed uncritically and in frightening excess.

Research into prescribing shows time and again that doctors will offer drugs when they are *not* the best solution to the patient's problems, and that they will prescribe when no treatment is necessary. Under these circumstances, there is not enough potential benefit to balance the unavoidable risk.

The cost of over-prescribing is not merely financial, though an NHS drug bill of £1,500,000,000 (1983) and rising is disturbing enough, but it also carries unmeasured costs in terms of drug-induced illness and the treatment necessary for its victims.

Doctors often fail to recognise adverse drug reactions for what they are, fail to report them to the Committee on Safety of Medicines, and fail to warn patients of the risks of drug therapy. Patients, for their part, are generally too eager to find an apparently easy solution to their health problems, preferring to rely on the doctor's prescription than to make positive effort on their own behalf.

We all need to be responsible for our own health, not off-loading responsibility onto doctors or the pharmaceutical industry. And one aspect of accepting responsibility is seeking information about treatment so that we can make rational choices.

It is always wise to ask your doctor questions about treatment, and about non-drug alternatives, and to follow up with visits to libraries to check reference books if you are thinking of taking any drug. There is a list of recommended sources at the end of this book.

With those provisos and warnings, let us consider what drugs are used for hay fever and what their use may involve.

The main thrust of medical effort is concentrated on relief of symptoms. Hay fever is not unusual in this respect; most illnesses are approached in this way. Something is done to ease the pain or remove the worst symptoms, while whatever caused the problem is largely ignored.

This may seem illogical, but we must remember that it is the symptoms, after all, that both doctor and patient are most aware of. So this is the obvious approach. The peculiar position of medicine as both an art and a science also tends to lead to less rigorous questioning of habits and assumptions among doctors. They spend less time than perhaps they ought trying to prevent disease.

There is no doubt that dealing with symptoms can bring welcome relief. In the case of hay fever, the easiest way to block the symptoms would be to stop the IgEs reacting and firing up the mast cells.

Because of the complex nature of the defence system involved, this has proved difficult. So medicine moved on a step, concentrating on ways to stop the worst effects of mast cell degranulation, and produced a variety of antihistamines.

Most hay fever sufferers who ask their doctors or pharmacists for help will be offered antihistamines. These drugs can eliminate the symptoms of hay fever completely in some very mild cases. But most people will need quite large doses, especially when the season is at its height, if they are relying on antihistamines alone. You will have to experiment to find out what suits you. It is advisable to take them after food to avoid potential stomach irritation. If a particular type of antihistamine is going to be of any use to you, you will notice the benefit within three days; there is no point in persisting for longer if there is no clear improvement.

The leading brand-name is Piriton, which can be bought in a variety of forms without a doctor's prescription. Usually, you'll get the little yellow 4mg tablets which can easily be cracked in half for precise control of the dose. There are many other forms of antihistamine, all with broadly similar effects; MIMS (the doctors' drug reference journal which lists the brands they can prescribe) included 22 different brand-names in the October 1983 edition, all recommended for hay fever, allergic conditions, or allergic rhinitis.

Two new antihistamines, Triludan and Hismanal, have different characteristics from the longer-established varieties. Animal experiments reveal that very little Triludan enters the brain, and neither product interacts with drugs such as Valium and alcohol to cause additional drowsiness and inco-ordination.

Side-effects recorded up to March 1984 include headache in some people who take Triludan, and occasional weight gain with Hismanal. Sedation is uncommon though not unknown. However, it is possible that serious adverse effects will come to light when these drugs have been in general use for longer. Anyone who takes either one and experiences any untoward reaction should report it to a doctor.

Triludan is now available without a prescription, but both these drugs are very much more expensive than the older antihistamines. Nevertheless, according to Merrell, the manufacturers, Triludan is now out-selling all other products in its class, so any dangers that it may have should come to light before very long.

As their name suggests, antihistamines work by blocking the effects of histamine. Every cell in the body is covered with what are called receptor sites. These enable the various chemical messengers, or mediators, to connect and convey their particular messages to the cell concerned. The cell will then carry out the function for which it was designed.

Antihistamines probably work by occupying the receptor sites where histamine would produce its effects on cells. They do not prevent the production of histamine or the degranulation of the mast cells caused by pollen in hay fever sufferers. Since mast cell degranulation produces far more than just histamine, a drug that blocks the effects of histamine and leaves most of the other products swilling around unaffected cannot be expected to provide complete relief.

Antihistamines do have other pharmacological actions which are largely independent of their effect on histamine receptors, but these seem to offer no advantage for hay fever sufferers.

They can antagonise or enhance the effects many of the other biochemical messengers — including acetylcholine, adrenaline, and serotonin — which have widespread actions throughout the body, but particularly in the nervous system.

This implies that they are capable of producing a rather unpredictable assortment of effects on mood, activity level, appetite, vision and all the other senses. The side-effects vary between individuals, and with the dose taken.

79

All but the newest antihistamines are known to cause drowsiness, they have a sedative effect. This is usually at low doses. Strangely at higher doses they can have the opposite effect, acting as stimulants.

The degree of sedation ranges from the imperceptible, through slight drowsiness, to deep sleep; and it can involve inability to concentrate, lassitude, dizziness, muscular weakness, and uncoordination. Other side-effects, experienced by a minority of users, include nausea, vomiting, diarrhoea or constipation, and stomach pain. Sometimes, they can cause headache, blurred vision, tinnitus (noises in the ears), elation or depression, irritability, nightmares, loss of appetite, problems with urination, dry mouth, and tingling, heaviness, and weakness of the hands.

Paradoxically, some highly susceptible people find that they become allergic to antihistamines. The allergy may be to some part of the carrier, or bulking agent in the pill, to the food colouring added to make it look distinctive, or, very occasionally, to the drug itself. Antihistamine *creams* are well known for producing allergic reactions, and most doctors avoid using them for that reason.

Used prudently, antihistamines are valuable drugs which can be taken to *complement* other measures. However, their sedative action can have serious consequences. It is so common that bottles containing antihistamine tablets or syrup are required by law to be dispensed with a label which warns, 'May cause drowsiness. If affected do not drive or operate machinery. Avoid alcoholic drink'.

While this warning is undoubtedly better than none, it does not go nearly far enough. Despite the drowsiness, antihistamines can give hay fever sufferers the illusion of being able to live a normal life. Consequently, the majority ignore the advice on the label.

A hay fever survey carried out for Merrell Pharmaceuticals in 1982 showed that 72% of drivers still drive while taking antihistamines; 78% of machinery operators still operate machinery; and 59% of those who normally drink alcohol continue to do so. It is predictable that those who do will be involved in accidents. This was confirmed by a study of motorbike crashes in Oxfordshire. Among those involved in motorbike accidents, there is a significant excess of people who have taken antihistamines.

In Norway the authorities take the risk of vehicle accidents so seriously that they require antihistamine bottles to carry a red warning triangle. This means that no one taking them is allowed to drive at all. Anyone who is caught driving while under the influence of antihistamines in Norway is liable to be imprisoned for up to a year.

Those who take any other drugs with sedative effects at the same time as antihistamines risk potentiation of the sedation, a much exaggerated degree of drowsiness. Alcohol is the most commonly used drug which has this characteristic, but the group includes tranquillisers, sleeping pills (which can linger in the body the day after they're taken), and some pain-killers including Distalgesic. It is also unwise to take antihistamines if you are also taking antidepressants.

Finally, we can only speculate on the potential consequences of interfering with our bodies' defences against infection by taking antihistamines.

It seems to us that such an approach must increase susceptibility to infection, but we know of no studies designed to test this hypothesis. However, our experience does lend support to the suggestion, for hay fever sufferers taking antihistamines do seem to catch more colds and develop more serious infections in the summer than at other times of the year.

For all this, we do not believe that hay fever sufferers should avoid antihistamines totally. Taken orally, they are relatively safe medicines. Our advice is that they should be used sparingly when safer alternatives have proved inadequate, and that those who take them should always be alert to the sort of problems that can arise with their use.

The second type of drug used to suppress hay fever symptoms is safer than antihistamine therapy, but has other disadvantages. It is a product which was originally developed for allergic asthma, but which has wide applications in other allergic disorders. This is sodium cromoglycate, sold under the brand-names Rynacrom, Lomusol, and Opticrom. Sodium cromoglycate can be obtained from a registered pharmacist without a doctor's prescription. But, unlike most antihistamines, it is expensive.

Sodium cromoglycate is capable of stabilising the membranes of the mast cells and preventing degranulation. It is believed to act by inhibiting the release of chemical mediators from sensitised mast cells, but other mechanisms may also be involved.

This drug must be applied directly and fairly frequently to the affected membranes, and it is ineffective once the allergic reaction has started.

To prevent the symptoms of hay fever in the nose, sufferers must begin to use Rynacrom (spray or drops) or Lomusol spray *before* the pollen to which they *expect* to react reaches the level at which symptoms start. They have to continue to use it for as long as they expect symptoms to be provoked.

If their eyes are affected, they will have to use Opticrom eye drops in the same way. And if the throat and bronchial tubes also react to pollen, they will need to use Intal (the same drug in a form designed for the treatment of asthma, available only on prescription), again before the hay fever season begins.

It is the people who use cromoglycate in any or all of its various forms who have most need of advance information about the pollen count. They have to take action against their symptoms before their bodies tell them that action is necessary. Fortunately for them, Fisons, the company that developed, manufactures and sells this drug, supports the National Hay Fever and Pollen Bureau. This organisation collects information about the weather and the soil temperature from 26 stations all over the country, and for the first time in 1983, it produced pollen forecasts to assist sufferers. Every day, from the beginning of the hay fever season in the south of England, to the end of it in the north of Scotland, local pollen counts are reported and pollen predictions worked out.

Anyone who uses sodium cromoglycate may be relieved to know that information about pollen counts can be obtained on Ceefax, the telephone weather service, breakfast TV, local radio, and many newspapers.

Only those membranes which are actually coated with the drug will be protected, so inaccessible parts of the body, like the eustachian tubes connecting the throat and the ear, cannot be treated.

Treatment with sodium cromoglycate has to be repeated frequently, up to six times a day. The drug is absorbed by the tissues in a matter of hours. However, the treatment is remarkably safe, because the drug is not broken down by the body at all but excreted unchanged. It seems not to have any effect except on those membranes to which it is applied. Its only known side-effect when used for the treatment of hay fever is local irritation. This is rare.

Many hay fever sufferers benefit from the use of sodium

cromoglycate, and those whose problems are restricted to the nose and eyes can become completely free of symptoms if they use the drug consistently. But for unknown reasons, it will not work for everyone, however carefully and regularly they douse their membranes. Different studies find widely varying rates of benefit, and there seems to be no way to predict which individuals can be helped by this drug.

The two approaches to symptomatic relief described above have the advantage of being fairly direct; the drug is aimed at the process of symptom production or its unwanted products. This is also a disadvantage, however. To work in this direct manner, the drug has to reach each seperate source of trouble.

In this, drugs have to be more effective than the pollen that triggers the reaction. If a comparatively small number of pollen grains fire up a few mast cells, this can be enough to produce widespread symptoms throughout the body. In the highly potentiated state in which the reaction occurs, other cells and bodily processes are readily persuaded to indulge in a chain-reaction of sympathetic response. Hence the sneezing and other symptoms elicited by pictures of flowers.

So any drug which is to counter symptoms in the most susceptible sufferers needs to have blanket coverage in order to stop any outbreak of reaction in the body. This is practically impossible to achieve.

In pursuit of a cure, medicine has been forced to approach the immune system and its hay fever malfunction from another direction. This is the third approach to symptom suppression with drug therapy, and it involves the use of synthetic forms of natural substances called steroids.

Steroids are produced in the body by the adrenal glands. Under natural conditions, they seem to be concerned primarily with the control of inflammation. They also have wide-ranging effects on metabolism. When we are involved in a strenuous physical activity such as running, the body produces adrenalin to make the muscles work harder, and steroids limit any localised inflammation that may occur as a result. If you were running for your life, it would be no good having to stop because of a blister on your foot or a sprained ankle.

When we are injured or subjected to any serious or lasting physical stress, steroids are produced. Their effects on the

83

metabolism lead to a rise in the blood sugar level, and generally keep the body in a fuelled-up state so that it is capable of dealing with any necessary activity and any problems that might be caused by that activity.

These actions are very roughly opposed to those of histamine. Histamines, as we saw, are part of a complex damage control system which is biased towards immobilising the body or parts of it to effect healing with the minimum of further damage. Steroids, on the other hand, are concerned with continued activity. They help the body to keep moving until it is out of danger.

To compensate for these potentially destructive effects, steroids then contribute to the healing process. They are dramatically effective in dealing with a wide variety of local problems, reducing irritation and soothing inflammation. Creams containing steroids will clear spots and rashes very quickly. But because they interfere with the normal functioning of the immune system, they increase chances of infection.

However, the other main effect of using synthetic steroids can be even more hazardous. In its attempts to return to a normal level of steroid in the system, the body cuts down on its own production. After a long term of steroid treatment, the adrenal glands will cease to produce natural corticosteroids, and eventually lose their ability to produce them.

Some of their many other dangers will be described later.

Synthetic steroids form the basis of a range of powerful drugs which used to be widely prescribed for hay fever. They can be taken by mouth, administered by injection, or applied directly to the membranes. They are only available on prescription.

The most frequently prescribed brands of nasal spray which include steroids are Beconase, Betnesol, Pabracort, and Syntaris. There are many different brands of systemic steroid (taken in a form which enters the whole body), but those which are offered in MIMS as suitable for hay fever are Betnelan and Betnesol tablets, and Acthar, Depo-Medrone, and Kenalog injections.

Steroids are highly effective drugs. They are capable of removing the symptoms of hay fever completely. This can be useful for severe sufferers who must be symptom free for special occasions such as weddings or crucial examinations, but if used for more than short periods they are *very dangerous*.

Fewer doctors now prescribe steroids for hay fever than

formerly. But the practice remains too common. Although some doctors imagine that steroid sprays applied to the nose do not carry the risks involved in systemic steroid therapy, there have been cases of severe damage induced by these products.

There is complacency about the use of steroid nose sprays, and patients are not given adequate warnings. Many doctors imagine them to be safer than they are.

The end result of careless repeat prescribing is personified by Babs Diplock, founder member of the Steroid Aid and Action Group. This brave and determined lady uses her own case as a living warning to other potential steroid victims.

Babs was working as a fish finger packer on Humberside when her job was threatened by hay fever. She was told, perhaps understandably, that she could not stay packing fish fingers unless she did something to control her running nose.

Her doctor prescribed cortisone, a highly effective drug. She was delighted, her hay fever was cured. She returned every year for sixteen years for injections, never dreaming that her doctor might be giving her a drug which could make her seriously ill.

Babs finally realised that something was going very wrong when her legs became so weak that she would fall down and be unable to get up. She had severe eye pain, high blood pressure, stomach pain, and pain in her bones. She became bloated, miserable, and at times suicidal. Her doctors prescribed more drugs to control the symptoms.

Four years later, Babs Diplock is somewhat improved, but she knows that she will never recover from the effects of steroids. Unfortunately she cannot stop taking them. Her adrenal gland no longer functions normally and does not produce enough corticosteroids for her to survive without replacement therapy. She treads a tightrope, taking as little steroid as she can, but just enough to stay alive.

The symptoms that Babs has described fall into the typical pattern of adverse reactions to steroids. They cause retention of water and sodium, high blood pressure, increased pressure inside the eye, and weakening of the bones which can result in spontaneous fractures and bone collapse.

Steroids may also induce diabetes and will certainly make it worse if you already have it. They interfere with wound healing, increase susceptibility to all types of infection, and can lead to the resurgence of infectious diseases such as tuberculosis from which a person had apparently recovered years earlier.

In children, they cause bones to mature before growth is complete, producing stunting and dwarfism.

And they can be absorbed through any tissues — including the skin, the nose, and the eyes.

The seriousness of their adverse effects means that steroids should only be used when there is *absolutely no alternative*. Perhaps predictably, they are overprescribed. Their effectiveness in controlling symptoms leads some patients to choose them rather than seek safer methods of dealing with their hay fever.

According to consultant allergist Dr Peter Borge, 'The use of long-acting steroids from April to June would most certainly lead to adrenal suppression'. This implies that controlling hay fever symptoms throughout one season with corticosteroids could lead to the failure of the systems on which we depend to cope with stress. When the adrenal glands fail to increase their output of steroids in response to physical stress, because of suppression due to drug therapy, the result can be collapse and death.

Anyone who has received corticosteroid therapy, by injection or by mouth, lasting for one month or more in any two-year period should carry a *warning card*, because collapse can occur during a surgical operation up to two years later.

There are some nose sprays which can be used for hay fever which contain neither sodium cromoglycate nor steroids.

Examples are Hayphryn, Otrivine-Antistin, and Vibrocil. Some sufferers use products which are not offered specifically for hay fever, but which share with these brands the ability to shrink the congested membranes of the nose.

Such products should be avoided. The only time to use them at all, and then for no more than a very short period, is when you have to cope with an emergency like an important interview. They contain drugs from a group known as sympathomimetics, which have actions which mimic those of adrenaline. They cause constriction of the small blood vessels.

Their most serious disadvantage is that they can cause 'rebound' congestion after use, so that the user needs to carry on using them or suffer an even stuffier nose. With repeated use, their effectiveness diminishes so that more and more is required. They can irritate the lining of the nose and in time they can produce permanent damage.

The same type of drug can be taken by mouth, and it is the active ingredient in some decongestants, such as Contac 400. Absorbed into the body, sympathomimetic drugs raise blood pressure, sometimes causing severe headache and potentially very serious hypertensive crises in vulnerable people. This is an idiosyncratic reaction; for unknown reasons, blood pressure rises dramatically in some people taking these drugs but not in others. If there is already blood vessel weakness, it could result in a stroke.

Because hay fever symptoms are long lasting, sufferers should not use any product whose main effect is just to reduce congestion in the nose. Their potential dangers outweigh the short-term benefits.

Use of all the products described above is aimed at *symptomatic relief*. In one way or another the drugs will suppress the symptoms. The objection to this form of treatment, aside from any hazards that may be involved in the use of each particular drug, is that you have symptoms because something basic is going wrong.

Symptoms are messages from your body. They should not be casually blanked off without at least understanding what they mean.

Perhaps the most apparently rational medical approach to hay fever is hyposensitisation (more commonly, but inaccurately, called desensitisation). This involves training the body to react less violently to particular allergens.

The groundwork for this type of treatment was carried out by a doctor working in the unit of St Mary's Hospital, Paddington, where Alexander Fleming studied penicillin. Dr Leonard Noon was following a tradition among doctors concerned with allergies, by doing research on himself. He was influenced by the homoeopathic approach to therapy, and chose to experiment with the very pollens to which he knew he was sensitive.

In 1911, Noon's paper describing his new type of treatment was published in the *Lancet*. His name is still used for the units of measurement of pollens and other allergens made up into hyposensitisation preparations.

Hyposensitisation is a long and relatively difficult procedure. It requires great care and skill because it carries potentially

87

serious hazards. However, when carried out by an experienced medical team, it can, according to enthusiasts, be very effective.

But the long-term effectiveness of hyposensitisation is controversial. There are others working in the field of allergy who maintain that it results in only a 50% reduction of symptoms in the average patient, and some end up worse than they began. Most studies report a success rate of around 70% — so between a quarter and a third of those who go through this unpleasant procedure are no better for it.

The question for the sufferer is whether the potential benefits are sufficiently great to balance the undoubted drawbacks. If the answer to this question is yes, the next problem is where to find a doctor who is capable of carrying out the procedure safely.

There are several steps in hyposensitisation. The first is to build up a very detailed case-history. A precise description of the dates of onset and cessation of hay fever will allow a tentative guess at the pollens responsible.

If you are considering hyposensitisation it makes sense to prepare for it by keeping a diary of your symptoms the season before you expect to go through the procedure. (Appendices I, II, V and VI will help here.)

In general, tree pollens cause the earliest problems, followed by grass and flower pollens, with fungal spores responsible for allergies in the autumn. At the same time, note whether you are most afflicted indoors or out, at what times of day, and under what circumstances. Many hay fever sufferers are also sensitive during the pollen season to house dust mite or animal hairs and other allergens (known as 'danders'), and may require hyposensitisation to these as well as to pollens.

All this information and more will go into the case-history. When this is complete, the allergist will have a good idea what is causing the allergy, but he or she will check these suspicions with a series of skin tests.

The most usual type of skin test is called the prick test. It involves dropping a very dilute solution of pollen or other potential allergen on the skin, usually the forearm, and pricking through the drop into the skin with a needle or lancet. This will be repeated for each suspected allergen. An allergic response will show up after 10 to 20 minutes as a white raised weal on an angry red flare as the local mast cells in the skin respond.

The problem with this test is that many people show sensitivity to allergens without suffering any symptoms. In the 20 to 30 year age group, one person in two will give a positive skin test to one of the commonest allergens — but only one in three of those who react is likely to develop hay fever.

There are other tests designed to check sensitivity to allergens, but some of these, such as nasal and bronchial challenge, are dangerous and offer no real advantage for diagnosis. There are laboratory tests; one of these involves counting the number of a particular sort of white blood cell, the eosinophil, which becomes more common in allergy. But eosinophil counts are too fallible to be of much use.

Unfortunately, skin tests are not always easy to interpret. Experience in judging the reaction is important, but there is still uncertainty because the size and appearance of the weal is not a perfect guide to the intensity of the allergic response. According to some experts, a positive reaction which develops in less than five minutes is evidence of high susceptibility. Doctors who fail to check the results of the test during this period will miss the significance of a fast reaction. However, the evidence for the importance of such signs is largely anecdotal and it may not be reliable.

It is important that sufferers do not take cough mixtures or other medicines containing antihistamines before a skin test.

After the allergens responsible for hay fever have been identified, as far as this is possible, treatment can begin with small doses of these substances. Hyposensitisation has to be carefully timed, to finish within a month of the onset of hay fever. If it continues into the beginning of the pollen season, it will make the condition worse, and the risk of a serious reaction is increased. And if it finishes more than three weeks before the season begins, its benefits can disappear.

A range of products are available for hyposensitisation. Most are 'tailor made' to match the results of the allergists' tests. The number of injections required will depend on the form in which the allergen is administered.

Bencard produce a comprehensive range of specific desensitising vaccines (SDV) for which an 18-injection course is usually required, as well as allergens in slow-release combinations (Alavac) which need to be given in nine to ten injections.

They also offer a three-dose system called Pollinex, in which the allergen is combined with the natural amino acid tyrosine. Pollinex is, predictably, the most popular product with general practitioners, but it is not individually tailored to each hay fever sufferer's needs. Nevertheless, it seems to be safer than some of the other forms. Other companies produce similar products in slightly different forms, for example Allpyral and Spectralgen.

Specific desensitising vaccines are normally given at weekly intervals, injected into the upper arm. These injections have to be given with great care. The doctor or nurse must be sure to avoid putting the vaccine between the skin layers or into a blood vessel.

Each dose is slightly higher than the last, and the assumption is that the body will adjust its tolerance level so that there will be no reaction to a concentration of pollens which would have induced allergy earlier in the course. If the injection causes anything more than a minor local reaction, it means that the concentration of allergen was too high and a smaller dose must be used for the next injection.

The risk with this procedure is that the injection can cause anaphylactic shock. If emergency treatment with adrenaline and oxygen is not given immediately, the outcome can be death. Nobody should commence hyposensitisation unless these facilities are readily available, and nobody who has had a hyposensitising injection should leave the clinic or doctor's surgery for at least twenty minutes — preferably half an hour — afterwards.

We heard from the mother of a young Plymouth trawlerman who was heartbroken about the way her son met his death. Michael had had fourteen injections of specific desensitising vaccine and set off 'in perfect health' for the fifteenth. The injection was given by a locum. When Michael complained that his hands felt peculiar and were losing their sensation, he was given an antihistamine tablet, and allowed to leave the health centre.

Michael staggered a short distance down the road before he collapsed. By chance he was taken back to the surgery by an off-duty ambulanceman. But he was already unconscious and an injection of adrenaline was not enough to revive him. No oxygen was available. Michael died just when the ambulance arrived to take him to hospital.

This case is far from unique. In a single volume of the *British Medical Journal* in 1980 (*281*, pp 854 and 1429), two cases of death after desensitisation treatment are described. In one, a nineteen-year-old girl with allergic asthma and rhinitis who had also received fourteen injections without reaction died after the fifteenth.

The first sign of a serious generalised reaction is usually itching, especially of the palms, followed by reddening of the eyes and a sensation of pressure in the ears. If this begins to happen, 0.5 ml. of adrenaline must be injected *immediately* near the site of the allergen injection, and repeated as often as necessary until the symptoms subside. Oxygen may also be necessary because the reaction can include the symptoms of severe asthma.

Hyposensitisation requires constant vigilance. If this is neglected, or if the doctor does not know how to treat a reaction or is unaware of the urgency of treatment, patients can and do die.

One of the many difficulties in this procedure is the way sensitivity to allergens varies from time to time. If a course of treatment is halted, with a gap of over three weeks in a series of weekly injections, the whole thing has to begin again. If the person receiving the treatment is suffering from an infection, the risk is greater, so the dose must be reduced.

These hazards are not the only drawbacks of this difficult procedure. Even after a course of injections, the allergic reaction may merely be reduced, not prevented; many people require courses on each of three successive years before they are free from hay fever, and even then, sensitivity is liable to return. They may need maintainence courses every other year for complete relief from symptoms.

Our advice is that anyone considering hyposensitisation treatment should go to a specialised allergy clinic where the method is well understood. In a few health centres, specially trained nurses and doctors who have a particular interest and experience in the use of this type of treatment can offer it with the minimum of risk. We would certainly not expect the average general practitioner to use hyposensitisation safely.

When every form of drug therapy has failed, some doctors will turn to other approaches. One is surgery, which in this case implies destruction of some of the tissue of the nose. This can only offer benefit if the main complaint is obstruction of the nose, and even those who have used some forms of surgery acknowledge that results of treatment are often unsatisfactory.

Both intense heat and cold have been used to destroy parts of the inside of the unfortunate victims' noses. One approach, submucosal diathermy, involves directing high-frequency electric currents to the tissue, effectively burning it away. Another involves applying a small but intensely cold probe to the swollen tissues (cryosurgery), which freezes the cells and kills them.

The Finnish practitioner who described this method admits that the reasons for its effectiveness are not known — though he claims very good results with up to seven monthly sessions of cryotherapy applied to the passages at the top of the nose. However, he also mentions that most of these patients had other forms of surgery too; and it is not clear who benefited from which treatment, or how long any benefit lasted.

One obvious drawback with any surgical approach is that it affects only a very limited area of tissue and thus could only be expected to offer local relief for some of the symptoms of hay fever.

Perhaps removal or destruction of the layer of mast cells lining the nose will prevent them from secreting for a while, but the body normally restores its integrity through extended growth of surrounding tissue. We would expect the problems to return, perhaps with additional unpleasantness due to scarring.

Modern technological approaches do not end here. Some hay fever sufferers have been exposed by enthusiastic practitioners to long wave ultraviolet radiation, others to laser treatment.

No doubt new approaches will continue to be developed as new machines become available. We would advise great caution before agreeing to submit to any treatment which is capable of causing irreversible damage.

Any form of treatment which involves physical alteration of parts of your body should be carefully considered in the light of your knowledge of the subtle systems involved. Even hyposensitisation, although apparently logical, does not really make much sense when *all* the factors involved in promoting the disease are taken into account.

Our opinion of the answers offered by conventional medicine is that they are of limited value because they do not address the nature of the problem and they are comparatively clumsy. They should be considered as very blunt instruments, and treated with due caution.

92

6 Alternative approaches

Alternative medicine (or complementary medicine, as it is sometimes called) has recently come into vogue. Even that most conservative of bodies, the British Medical Association, now accepts its importance. One reason for its new popularity is undoubtedly disenchantment with conventional approaches to the treatment of ill health, because of their hazards and the emphasis on palliation.

However, responsible alternative practioners are now becoming concerned that alternative methods are being misused in much the same way as conventional medicine has been. The basic principles of rational therapy are just as important in alternative medicine; and the fact that a particular pill is made with herbs does not necessarily make it safer or more effective than its synthetic counterpart.

While it makes little sense to require that alternative medicine prove itself in tests more stringent than any applied to conventional medicine, it is not rational to reserve our scepticism for one approach while accepting uncritically the dictates of another.

Alternative medicine has fewer controls than conventional medicine largely because its dangers are less. However there are those who, having become disenchanted with their conventional doctors, then go the rounds of the alternatives and are treated no better.

There are practitioners who peddle nonsense at a high price. There are books proposing diets and regimes that are more likely to do harm than good.

The essential lesson is that we cannot drop our guard and off-load responsibility for health onto those whose magic pills and potions are made from seaweed or curious concoctions of plants, if the fundamental approach — take this and you will magically recover — is exactly the same, and likely to be equally erroneous.

That said, there can no longer be any reasonable doubt that some alternative types of treatment which had for decades been dismissed as rubbish by the medical establishment *are* effective.

Homoeopathic remedies which should, according to conventional theory, have no effect on anything, have been demonstrated to produce reliable effects on the growth of plants and yeasts under controlled laboratory conditions. Acupuncture has been demonstrated to produce on rats in prestigious Western university laboratories the effects observed by the ancient Chinese. Hypnosis is no longer confined to crank practitioners and showmen, but researched by psychologists and used in many areas of therapy.

A wide variety of treatments for hay fever is offered by alternative practitioners. Some of these are also available from the growing number of NHS doctors who have been trained in alternative systems. Those who want to try one of these may be able to persuade their G.P.s to refer them to NHS clinics where alternative approaches are used, for example at the homoeopathic hospitals in London, Glasgow, Liverpool and Bristol.

Those who search their local health/wholefood shop for remedies for hay fever are likely to find herbal catarrh remedies, mineral preparations, and homoeopathic remedies.

They may also find books which offer advice on the treatment of hay fever by an assortment of means. Some of this advice is sensible and will probably improve the general health of the sufferer; however, this is not true of all of it.

We were very dubious, for example, about the value of Alan Moyle's *Nature Cure for Asthma and Hay Fever*. Mr Moyle believes that asthma and hay fever are primarily caused by poor diet — particularly an excess of cooked carbohydrate and protein and the drinking of tea and coffee — and that most people 'depend on a series of colds, catarrh, acne and other eliminatory flare-ups to expel accumulated poisons'. The impression given is that hay fever is one of these eliminatory flare-ups.

The treatment proposed includes fasting followed by semi-starvation, enemas, and cold baths in a variety of forms. While his general comments on dietary improvements are fairly sensible, we would not agree that fasting for five days or more and subsistance on the strictly limited regime he proposes for an unspecified period thereafter would be likely to benefit the health of the majority of people; indeed, it could be dangerous. We are equally unhappy about cold baths. As for enemas, we would warn readers that they too can be risky if used often, and they are quite unnecessary for the majority of people.

This brings us to a general point. If any treatment for hay fever were reliably effective for every sufferer who used it, we could reasonably expect that that treatment would have developed a strong reputation, and that it would have imitators. We could find no evidence of any such phenomenon, nor anyone who, offering a range of alternatives, was confident that one in particular would be reasonably certain to work. There seems to be no consensus, outside the medical world, on how hay fever should best be treated.

Whether the various herbal mixtures we have seen on sale would benefit many hay fever sufferers, we do not know. Neither have we been able to discover any reliable evidence that mixtures made up by specialised herbalists for individual sufferers are likely to be helpful, and we can therefore offer no judgement on them. The same applies to tissue salts, biochemic remedies, and the like. We would be interested in any carefully controlled clinical trials of these remedies.

If you have *faith* in one of these alternative systems, then the probability that it would work for you is higher than if you are totally sceptical. The strength of the patient's commitment to the therapeutic regime has been shown in research studies to be one of the strongest determinants of the placebo effect — the ability of inactive medicines to cure illness or reduce symptoms.

Placebos are medicines containing no active ingredients which have nevertheless been conclusively demonstrated to produce therapeutic effects.

They are capable of enhancing the power of the individual's own healing systems. They are important in every type of medicine because the patient plays a crucial part in the therapeutic process: he or she is far more than a passive recipient of the doctor's ministrations. If patients believe that, far from doing good, the treatment will harm them, then negative placebo effects can operate to reduce or reverse the therapeutic value of the treatment. In fact, this phenomenon is well recognised in conventional medicine; some surgeons, for example, are extremely reluctant to operate on patients who believe they will die as a result — because these patients *do* die far too often.

Hay fever is an excessive and inappropriate reaction of the individual's immune system. In theory, at least, it must be possible for the reaction to be corrected from within, so that the individual recovers completely from the condition. This, presumably, is what happens when spontaneous remission takes place.

So it is quite feasible for some type of treatment which might in itself have no justification by current scientific or medical standards to produce a total or partial cure, if that treatment had such a powerful impact on the sufferer that he or she was inspired to recover.

It is most unlikely that a bottle of tablets bought in the local health store would have this sort of impact. But a remedy selected individually for the sufferer by a sympathetic and trusted herbalist or other practitioner with great personal magnetism could well work. *How* it works does not, after all, matter greatly to the sufferer. In fact, controlled trials of hay fever treatments regularly show a high placebo effect.

The most powerful form of this type of effect is, of course, 'faith healing', or healing by laying on of hands, which does not require the use of any medication or other aid. Those sceptics who insist on denying the value of this type of healing must be more concerned with holding on to their own prejudices than with looking into the evidence, for effective healers have been active throughout history, all over the world. But we would not advise such sceptics to consult faith healers in their search for a cure for hay fever — we would expect the treatment to fail for them.

Those who benefit from their experience with healers usually report a sensation of heat or tingling or both, emanating from the healer's hand and penetrating deeply into their bodies, drawing away any pain. We have not heard about the use of this type of healing for hay fever in particular, but there is some evidence of success with asthma.

Acupuncture is another type of healing with roots that go back into early history. Chinese manuscripts dealing with acupuncture date from 2,500 years ago. How it works, in western terms, is not known. The eminent psychologist Professor Ron Melzack has developed a theory that partially explains its effectiveness for pain relief but his explanation would not imply that acupuncture could help hay fever sufferers. However, there is strong evidence that it can reduce the allergic response.

While scientists strive and largely fail to explain acupuncture in terms of their own particular disciplines, the system holds little mystery for traditional practitioners who accept a different way of looking at the body and its processes.

According to traditional Chinese theory, vital energy — *Chi* — circulates around the body along channels known as meridians. There are twelve principal meridians, ten of which are associated with different organs of the body, and two corresponding to 'functions'. In addition, there are meridians running along the midpoint of the body, one at the front and one down the spine.

The acupuncturist's task is to ensure that *Chi* flows along these channels properly. He diagnoses faults in the flow by feeling the pulse at the wrists, where the state of the meridians can be judged. He will then correct these faults by inserting needles at crucial points along the appropriate meridians and manipulate them to stimulate the chosen points.

Recent technological advances have provided acupuncturists with new ways of stimulating these points, some of which do not require the use of needles. Acupressure — stimulation by pressing or rubbing — is the best known. In China and in the West, the needles may be wired up to an electrical stimulator. Traditionally, they are twisted rapidly by hand.

A careful study of acupuncture therapy for allergic rhinitis was reported in the *American Journal of Chinese Medicine*. The authors referred to other research — in Czechoslovakia, China, and Indonesia — which also showed that acupuncture could be beneficial for the majority of sufferers.

Twenty-two sufferers, average age 34 years, were given six sessions of acupuncture, and their symptoms declined steadily throughout the treatment. By the end of the sixth session, half the group were virtually free of symptoms, eight (36%) had reduced symptoms, and three (14%) were no better. There were no adverse reactions, nor did any patient report worse symptoms after the treatment.

After two months, 36% had suffered partial relapse, but the

majority showed lasting benefits — improvements which were confirmed by laboratory tests showing reduced IgE and eosinophil levels. The implication of this is that acupuncture is capable of reducing general allergic susceptibility but, like so many therapeutic approaches to hay fever, it does not work for everybody.

To our knowledge, the only other alternative treatment for hay fever which has been tested in a carefully-designed scientific study is homoeopathy.

This is the therapeutic system developed by Samuel Hahnemann, an eighteenth-century German doctor who was so horrified by the medical practices of his day that he vowed never to subject his patients to such torture. At that time, it was fashionable to use so-called 'heroic' measures on the unfortunate sick. Bleeding was often so frequent and prolonged that patients would be left with no strength to fight disease; blisters were applied to the skin, causing painful sores; concoctions of toxic drugs were given in such quantities that patients were regularly poisoned by them. Only the supremely fit could withstand such treatment, the sick had little chance.

Hahnemann studied chemistry, developing an unusually detailed knowledge of the substances used in the preparation of medicines. Ever mindful of the ancient medical dictum *Non nocere* — do no harm — he set about investigating the effects of *minimal* quantities of these drugs.

His research convinced him that toxic substances had healing powers in very low concentrations; and that the particular healing effect of each closely paralleled its effects in higher concentrations. From this evidence he developed the idea that like could be used to treat like: in other words, that to cure a particular set of symptoms he should use a remedy that, in higher doses, would produce identical symptoms.

With his students, he compiled a list of the symptom picture induced by each of hundreds of different substances. Since Hahnemann's first books appeared in the early nineteenth century, the list has been extended by his successors so that virtually every poison is now available in the minute doses employed by homoeopaths.

Homoeopathic medicines are produced in a range of

'potencies', but in contrast to other systems, the higher potencies actually contain *smaller* quantities of the original substance. They are produced by successive dilution of a solution containing the basic substance, with agitation ('succussion') at each step. After many dilutions, a single dose of the final preparation may actually contain none of the original substance from which it was prepared.

What remains is, in effect, an impression left on the surrounding molecules by the original substance.

Doctors trained in conventional science have long denied the possibility that a substance that cannot be detected by any chemical means can have a therapeutic effect. So, to answer these critics, some homoeopathic doctors have carried out experiments designed to show that these high potencies *do* have biological effects. At the London Homoeopathic Hospital, Dr Michael Jenkins has demonstrated that some of the most widely-used remedies produce reliable, if not totally explicable, effects on the growth of yeasts and wheat seedlings.

At the homoeopathic hospital in Glasgow, Dr David Taylor Reilly and his wife Morag, a scientist, chose the treatment of hay fever as a test of the effectiveness of the method. A pilot study revealed a marked reduction in the symptoms experienced by hay fever sufferers who took mixed grass pollens in a dose so small (30 c potency) that the pills may not have contained any pollen at all. Patients were given homoeopathic pills or sugar pills prepared to look and taste exactly the same, and neither doctor nor patient knew whether the code on the packet meant that the pill contained an active substance or not. An 'escape therapy' of antihistamine treatment was available to those hay fever sufferers whose symptoms were unacceptably severe.

At the end of the study, when the results had been collected, the code was broken by the experimenters. The results showed that the patients taking the real medicine experienced a 75% reduction in overall symptoms, as compared with a 15% reduction in patients taking the dummy treatment. This is astonishingly high by any standards. And, in contrast to conventional medical treatments, there were no side-effect problems. Those involved in the study hope to repeat it on a larger scale in 1984, so that the value of this type of treatment can be conclusively demonstrated.

Dr Reilly did not plan his study primarily as a homoeopathic clinical trial of the use of mixed grass pollens in the treatment of hay fever. It was intended merely to show that these incredibly dilute medicines could affect the course of illness. Nor does he believe that this is necessarily the ideal homoeopathic treatment for all sufferers.

Homoeopathy offers three basic ways of dealing with hay fever. The first is the 'local' approach, which involves the use of remedies which, in large doses, produce a pattern of symptoms similar to hay fever. One ingredient of such a remedy might be *Allium cepa* — a particularly eye-watering variety of Spanish onion. Euphrasia (Eyebright) and Sabadilla, which causes sneezing, are also used in this way. These ingredients are present in most homoeopathic hay fever remedies which are available over the counter in some chemists' and health shops.

Dr Jenkins has not found the local approach to be of much value in hay fever. He uses less well-known remedies, particularly potencies of allergens of the type tested in the Glasgow study.

This is the second type of therapy, and it has much in common with immunisation, except that the doses are very much smaller than those used in any other system of treatment.

Interestingly this closely parallels the use by clinical ecologists of minute doses of food allergens to protect sufferers from reactions. One clinical ecologist's comment on this similarity was that 'clinical ecology is proving the veracity of homoeopathy'!

The third approach is the one that is most generally used in homoeopathy. Prescribing is based on an overall picture of the individual patient. It requires a long and detailed interview designed to elicit information about every aspect of the individual. The homoeopath aims to improve the general functioning of the patient and correct whatever imbalance may have led to the production of symptoms.

This is the 'constitutional' approach, and it is very close to the concept of holistic medicine. Holistic medical practitioners not only seek to have a whole view of individuals as persons, but also to relate those persons to their environment in a dynamic way. This means taking account of the interaction both within and outside, balancing the personal processes with those of the wider environment.

The homoeopathic approach to hay fever seems to involve gently persuading the immune system of its error. By correcting all the related factors that the practitioner may perceive, the body meets the allergen when all is relatively calm. With luck it will not react. Something like stroking a wild dog rather than cuffing or kicking it.

The results may not be instant, but the method is safe. It might take two or three years of perseverance before the body is persuaded that pollen is not harmful. Even then a small quantity of antihistamine, or a course of homoeopathic potencies of pollens, might be necessary at the worst time of the year. While you still live in the same environment you are still subject to the same influences, and it might be expecting too much for your body not to respond to the stress at all.

Clearly, it is not possible to conduct a controlled trial of the remedies used by practitioners who prefer the third approach. Each hay fever sufferer would require a different treatment, and any change in the level of hay fever symptoms would be just one of a range of possible effects. This approach could also be expected to produce a high rate of placebo effects, but how beneficial any other therapeutic effects might be is bound to be questionable from the sceptic's standpoint.

To summarise, then, two forms of alternative treatment for hay fever have been shown in carefully designed trials to be beneficial. These are acupuncture and homoeopathy, the latter using high (i.e. extremely dilute) potencies of specific allergens — in this case, mixed grass pollens. Neither has the drawbacks of serious side-effects or adverse drug reactions, and we would therefore suggest that hay fever sufferers seek out trained practitioners in these fields and try them.

Regrettably, as with conventional medicine, not all those who offer treatment are actually competent to use the systems of therapy on which they rely.

Neither system can be expected to work for every hay fever sufferer, but both have shown good results for the majority.

Other types of alternative therapy, including such things as aromatherapy and reflexology, may well work for some, but there is a dearth of convincing evidence demonstrating their effectiveness in the treatment of hay fever. We must leave to individual judgement the decision of whether they are worth trying.

7   Action summary

Hay fever is a true environmental disease. Its causes are predominantly in our environment, and any permanent relief from its effects will result from modifying those causes.

The use of any medication involving risk should be regarded as a last resort. Drugs should be taken only when all else has been tried, or circumstances are sufficiently dire to justify the risk. The apparent convenience of drugs, whether bought over the counter or prescribed by a doctor, is not really adequate justification. Too many hay fever sufferers spend every year on the pill treadmill, trying first this one, then that one, and finding that none provide a satisfactory answer.

Reducing your hay fever suffering to the absolute minimum may take a little time. It was probably a number of years before the disease got to the stage where it became an identifiable complaint. It is only reasonable to expect to take perhaps two or three years to get rid of it. Instant cures are very rare with any long-term disease.

But there are steps you can take immediately to start you on the road to improvement.

When following any measure to improve your health it is important that you try to tune in to what is actually happening to you. The feedback you give yourself is the best guide to the effectiveness of your actions.

The rules are simple: if it feels good, or better, do a little more, if it has no effect try something else, if it makes you worse, work out why, and avoid it.

Any action you take will be more beneficial if you have a strongly positive attitude towards what you are doing. Half hearted measures tend to get less than half hearted results, so make up your mind that you have had enough of hay fever, and you are now going to avoid it.

Get your family or friends to join in. After all they have to put up with you being irritable or half asleep for most of the summer, so your success is clearly to their advantage as well. Make it a joint effort. Many of the suggestions below would be better followed in company.

Positive action for hay fever sufferers must take account of the time of year. To allow for this we have split the action into three parts. First there are things you can do all the year round. If you are now in the middle of your hay fever season, perhaps you should start with the second part, headed 'In the season'. The most important time for decisive action, however, is out of season, perversely at that time when we would rather forget all about it. This is the time when you can tinker with your body, should you decided to do so, with minimum risk.

And it is also the time of year when you are free of those symptoms that inhibit action when the pollen is about. Make the most of it so that when the pollens return they will have less effect on you.

All The Year Round

Improve your general health. There are very few people who would not benefit from this, and because the British are so generally unfit, the benefit from a small change is often disproportionately large.

We live in bodies designed for action, but the way we live frequently acts against this fact. The motor car has wasted our legs away, and with them the capacity of our heart and lungs. To many people the thought of walking a couple of miles, or running a few hundred yards, is a terminal proposition.

No matter what age you are, you will benefit from more activity. Even those who are on the go all day and come home exhausted will feel better for a little extra exertion of another type. Doing more increases your capacity to do more, so the normal activities of the day, rather than taking you to your limit, come well within your capacity.

If you are a nervous or hyper-active type, try following your activity with a period of meditation or yoga relaxation exercises to redress the balance. Learn to switch off as well as on. But you will tend to find that physical activity will tend to reduce mental over-activity.

103

And there is no need for the thought of special equipment or expensive facilities to stop you. You can start right now with what you have got — yourself!

If you are *very* inactive, overweight or elderly, a good start might be to put on a favourite piece of music, one that really takes you somewhere else, and spend as long as it takes to move and stretch every part of your body. Let the music take you as you discover yourself. *Really* stretch and move, though, don't doze off.

Next, the simplest thing to do is to walk. Not stroll, or amble, but walk. Try to imitate the very brisk pace of the Durham Light Infantry. Start off with three sessions a week, at any time to suit yourself, with a day off in between. When you go for your walk, wear sensible shoes such as trainers (otherwise you will be learning about the biochemistry of blisters in a painful way) and warm loose clothing.

Then set off at a cracking pace, shoulders back, arms swinging and breathing deeply and easily. It does not matter if at first you cannot keep it up for long. Brisk minutes are much better than sloppy hours.

One word of caution about all forms of unaccustomed exercise. Overdoing it is as bad as underdoing it. Do enough to *feel* the effort, then stop, relax completely, have a warm bath. Your metabolism will be working on the effects of your exercise for the next twenty-four to forty-eight hours.

When you have got to the stage when you can walk briskly for an hour, covering between four and six miles, three times a week, you should start running.

You could go to dance classes, do aerobics, play tennis, follow any *active* sport. Very overweight people should choose a form of activity where their weight is supported; if they increase the activity level, gradually that weight will come off. But in the meantime, to avoid putting too much strain on the joints, the best sports for them are swimming and cycling.

Use your battle against hay fever to do those things you have hankered towards for years. Whatever activity you pursue, make sure it has some strenuous content. And of course running is the way to stay fit for any sport. So. . . .

You will need running shoes, and a track suit, and possibly a sweat band. Fit people need these things, and you are well on your way to being fit. Running is the one activity that beneficially affects nearly all bodily systems. It is what we were designed to do!

Now, do not get misled into jogging. It is not the same thing as running. Joggers plod along at a constant rate, a little above walking speed (your new walking speed) and believe they are doing good. When running, you should vary your speed throughout your hour session.

At first you will run a little, and walk a lot. Don't worry about this, there's no point injuring yourself by expecting too much too fast. Run until you are breathless — not too fast at first — and then walk till you have recovered and can run a bit more. When you are doing more running than walking, then vary the pace, do some sprinting, amaze yourself with your speed! Running continuously for an hour, you will be impressed with your own stamina.

It might take you two or three years to get to that stage, depending on how old and unfit you are. But the improvement it will make in *all* areas of your life will make the effort well worthwhile.

And you can either do it on your own, or get all your friends and family involved. Impromptu running groups are springing up in many places. The London 'Hash Hound Harriers' manage to carefully plan a gallop to suit all abilities from a pub to another pub during Sunday lunchtimes. If there isn't a group, why not start one?

Some people who run manage to carry on smoking. Most do not. Giving up smoking in isolation is very difficult, but as part of a goal orientated approach to life it is easier. Get serious about your running or sports ability and smoking will get in the way and have to go.

Giving up smoking is probably the best single move you could make to improve your health.

We are well aware of the difficulties in giving up. We are both ex-smokers. What you need more than anything else is total determination *not* to let nicotine prove itself to be more powerful than your will. The benefits will become apparent quickly; those who are prone to respiratory problems of any sort find that their susceptibility falls within weeks of ceasing to irritate their membranes with cigarette smoke.

The probability that you fall victim to any cold or flu virus that's around will drop to about half of its previous level, and reducing susceptibility to infection will reduce the severity of your hay fever.

As with all other aspects of health promotion, giving up smoking is much easier with social support. Get the whole household to work with you in a joint effort to quit; that way, you all benefit. Partners could try having sex instead of a cigarette, this 'threat or promise' approach may stimulate your efforts, and it is definitely healthier.

Just as we were never meant to be inactive smokers, we were not designed to live on the typical British diet. The ideal diet contains as much untreated food as possible, especially fruit and vegetables — you can't eat too much of this type of food. Cereals and grains are excellent too, but they must not be milled to produce the fine white substitute that we find too often in our supermarkets. Wholemeal bread, brown rice, wholemeal pasta, and other whole foods really do have more nourishment and more flavour than the processed white forms.

Have you ever stopped to wonder why the junk food merchants have to add so many flavourings, texturisers, sweeteners, colourings, odourisers and other additives to their products? The reason is simple — all the natural flavour and texture have been removed from the product. Pigs and cattle are fed on it because it's very nutritious. That way, the cereal merchants can sell the same grain twice. Why should you co-operate with that?

If you increase the proportion of natural fruit and vegetable products in your diet, you will be automatically correcting the major flaws. Most people in Britain would benefit by reducing the quantity of animal products (meat, butter, animal fat) they eat, cutting out all sugar except what is naturally present in fruit, and cutting back on sodium in the form of salt, baking powder, 'flavour enhancers', etc.

Work at it gradually. Improving a family's eating habits can take a long time. If you try one change a week you will move steadily in the right direction.

Having set out on this course of improving yourself and your diet, you should look to your immediate environment, and remove all unnecessary substances that might contribute to your allergy problem.

The kitchen and bathroom are two of the most concentrated sources of allergens. Be ruthless with sprays — if possible, chuck them all in the bin. You can live without them and they cause damage to your delicate membranes. Review your chemical cleansers and polishes, and chuck as many away as you can bear. And don't replace those that run out if there is an alternative. You don't want any avoidable chemicals in your air.

In some parts of the home, we don't recommend the use of natural substances. The reason is that the ubiquitous house dust mite, to which very many people are especially sensitive in the hay fever season, thrives in such items as feather pillows. Feather bedding has been described as a 'luxuriant breeding ground for the continuous growth and proliferation of household mites', by an American allergist. Out with it.

If the mites don't bother you, the fungi which also prefer natural fibres may. Take a thorough look at your bedroom: could moulds be flourishing there? They like damp conditions, one of the favoured creations of British house builders for many decades. There may not be a simple answer, but the possibility is worth investigating.

To reduce the level of mites to the minimum, you should remove all their favourite breeding-places. These include carpets, spring interior mattresses, and soft toys. Ideally, the allergy-prone person's bedroom should be rather spartan, with wooden floors, and a minimum of fabric. Foam rubber mattresses have been shown to harbour a mere one third of the number of mites found in spring mattresses!

While you are still free of hay fever, and considering your home, why not adapt the house — or at least, the part that you occupy for the largest proportion of the time — to create a pollen-free haven?

The room most worth pollen-proofing will be one of the coolest in the house, because you won't want it to get too hot in there when the windows are sealed shut on sunny days. So it's likely to be downstairs. Double glazing and thick curtains will help if the sun does shine in.

It is important that the door should fit well, and that everybody in the household should get used to leaving it shut. This door and the next one between your haven and the outside world should be both kept shut as much as possible.

Going out to work can be difficult. Despite many years of pressure and agitation many people are still forced to work in conditions that are far from healthy. Pressure of numbers, particularly out of work numbers, will ensure that this remains a difficult topic. Even more so when workers are forced to compete with their third world equivalents, and the office staff are threatened by the power of the microchip.

Under these circumstances it is paradoxical that work is increasingly valued for its social content. This fact may enable specific groups like hay fever sufferers (two may constitute a group) to apply pressure for improvements in the conditions or environment that will ease their problem, and make them more effective as employees. Press for a smoke and pollen free work place.

Going out brings us to the great outdoors.

It is the generalised industrial pollution that is your enemy here. This is the root cause of hay fever as we know it. There may be little you can do about it as an individual, and you may be the sort of person who just wants to remove the personal effects of the problem, and not worry too much about its effect on others.

But there are people who are concerned about pollution.

It is regrettably true that the British authorities do not have a good record of fast action to protect subjects from environmental hazards. It seems to be necessary to give all benefits of doubt to the industry or institution involved, rather than to the public. Organisations do exist to bring pressure to bear to change this; they range from groups concerned with specific issues, such as lead in petrol, or asbestos, to general action groups like Greenpeace, and alternative political parties, such as the Greens in Germany, and the Ecology Party in Britain.

All of these groups are minorities, but perhaps you should consider helping or joining them. Their motivation is concern for life and health.

In The Season

During the pollen season, your first task is to find out as much as you can about your hay fever and the pollens that trigger it. You will need to keep a detailed diary. (See Appendices.)

Record in your diary the severity of the symptoms you suffer from the day they begin. If the spring was warm and sunny, that day will tend to come earlier than after a damp, cold spring.

Note carefully the times when your symptoms are at their worst, and anything that seemed to precipitate them, whether at work or in the home. This will help you to discover your triggers, and allow you to take avoiding action.

Make a note, also, for the prevailing weather conditions each day. An overcast morning followed by a bright afternoon will tend to delay the production of pollens by grasses, for instance. The pollen count, announced in the media, should also be recorded; it may or may not be a good predictor for you, but you need to know.

Over the course of a week or two, patterns will start to emerge from the notes in your diary. Then you can adapt your activities according to all the signs that predict the severity of symptoms.

If, despite your attempts to avoid pollen, your symptoms become severe, you may want to damp them down with drugs. But it is worth using just the mimimal quantity of medication, because blotting symptoms out completely not only entails risk of drug problems, but it is bound to interfere with your longer term task of getting to understand your hay fever.

Even if your hay fever is in full spate, you can try some of the alternative medical approaches to treatment. Homoeopathic levels of grass pollens can be effective, as can acupuncture.

If you can get away from your allergic triggers completely during the worst of the hay fever season, then that is clearly what you should do. If June is normally your worst month take your holiday then, and head south to the Mediterranean, or out to sea. Don't worry about the heat making you even more miserable — just make sure you're far enough south for the grass to have ceased flowering, or for the weeds that set you sneezing to be left behind in the temperate zone.

A century ago, Blackley recommended an ocean voyage or a period on a small island a long way from land; his advice is as sensible now as it was then — for those who can afford to follow it!

If you can't go as far as the Mediterranean, then head for the southern resorts of the West Country, or the West coast of Ireland, or Brittany in France where the prevailing winds blow from the sea. But beware! Choose your spot carefully, and *don't go camping.* The seaside won't be any more comfortable than inland if the wind blows over meadows near the coast, and you'll not have your pollen-proof room to go to.

At home it may be a good idea to sleep in your pollen-proof room at the height of the season. This may also be the time and place to experiment with an ionizer.

Out Of Season

This is the time for serious action. If you have not been through a pollen session and written a detailed diary of your symptoms, try to make notes from memory of the things suggested above for your diary.

You will need this information in as detailed and accurate a form as you can get it if you are considering any form of hyposensitisation.

You will particularly need this information if you are going to a homoeopath to try to prevent your trigger firing up your mast cells. This is the approach we would recommend. Unfortunately there are relatively few homoeopaths working inside the NHS, so it may mean paying for a private consultation.

After trying almost everything conventional medicine had to offer, the £22 we spent with a South Wales homoeopath was the best deal ever. In the first year of treatment symptoms were reduced by 50%, and the same in the following year. By year three, the hay fever problem had practically disappeared.

Although acupuncture is more directly concerned with modifying processes in action, out of season may be the time to start looking for a practitioner if you are considering this therapy. They are even fewer in number than homoeopaths, and establishing contact well in advance of need would be wise.

With any treatment it is important to establish clear communication with the person treating you. This is particularly true of holistic treatments where you are being considered as a complete entity. In these situations the more empathetic the relationship between you, the better chance you have of achieving good results. Any doctor or healer who will not communicate with you should be regarded as suspect.

If you are considering hyposensitisation by conventional methods it is essential that you discuss it fully with the practitioner you are consulting. Write a check list from the points raised in chapter Five, take it with you, and note down the answers you are given. Only if you are completely satisfied on every point should you go ahead, and then you must watch very carefully for signs of problems.

Our categorical advice would be to first seek help from a homoeopath, then possibly an allergist. Only as a matter of last resort, and if your hay fever is unbearable, should you consider hyposensitisation at a specialised clinic.

We cannot say too often that whichever measure you opt for, the results will be enhanced by an improvement in your general health. Go back to the beginning of this chapter and run through the actions suggested. Keep doing this until you convince yourself that you cannot go on without being a much healthier person!

And keep firmly in your mind the question of the major cause of hay fever, industrial pollution. While improving your general health, and tackling your personal hay fever problem, do something to improve our shared environment.

Environmental disease has a political dimension. Those who watch and wait while millions become *avoidably* ill have failed to live up to the trust society has placed upon them. Whether they are politicians or health professionals, until they cease offering cures, and instead seek to remove the *causes* of such sickness they will continue to fail.

Medicine in our society is devoted to the concept of cure, not prevention. Therefore you must accept the responsibility for *maintaining* your health, and live your life in accordance with the demands of that responsibility. You will find it rewarding in practice.

Good luck, and good health!

THE END

Postscript

We wrote this book shortly after returning to live in London from rural South Wales where we had spent the previous five years. As our research on the causes of hay fever proceeded I began to wonder if the move had been a bad mistake.

Sure enough, in the spring of 1984, amid the polluted city air, the symptoms which had disappeared in the meadows and forests of Wales re-emerged. Those pollutants were pushing my systems once more beyond their limits and into over-load and reaction. True, it was not as bad as it had been before, just minor irritation, I could still run in the evenings and carry on working. But it was a warning — if I subjected myself to city pollution hay fever would be the inevitable result.

Two things happened to help me avoid this. First, I rigorously applied the recommendations in this book to myself, then to boost my general health further I followed a detailed personal programme developed by Life Profile Ltd. (A company for which we now work, adding to the information it provides to clients via a system of computerised analysis and development of personal health programmes.) This action held the problem at bay in the city. Secondly, at the end of the summer, we moved out to rural Suffolk. Once more we are surrounded by plant life. Next spring I do not anticipate any problem with hay fever.

I hope you have been able to learn enough about your condition and situation to say the same.

Colin Johnson, October 1984.

Useful books to read

One of our reasons for writing this book was the discovery that there was no comprehensive book on hay fever for the ordinary reader.

This is not to say that books have not been written on the subject. Many have. But they all seem to limit themselves to steering the reader more or less directly to a particular belief or remedy, with little attempt at giving either understanding of the disease or choice of action in dealing with it.

For these reasons we have not felt able to include any of the other hay fever books we have discovered in our reading list. If there is a good one, we are sorry we have not been able to find it and recommend it to you.

There is, however, a wide-ranging prize-winning essay on the subject written by Dr R.W. Harland and published in the *Journal of the Royal College of General Practitioners* (1979, *29*, 265–286).

The books we have listed below are ones that we have found either helpful or interesting in coming to grips with the problem. They deal with background topics, and we hope they will add to your understanding of your condition.

What On Earth Are We Doing? Ladybird Books. A beautiful illustrated environmental primer, aimed at children. We would give this book to everyone as a present if we could. There is no reason why kids should not share the good things. Highly recommended.

Silent Spring by Rachael Carson (1962). A popular classic of early environmental awareness.

The Picture of Health by Erik Eckholm (1977). A wide view of the determinants of health. Discusses medicine and environmental factors and includes numerous examples relating the effects of everyday things to the whole picture.

Our Chemical Environment by Murray Bookchin (1962). A pioneering overview of the problems of artificial chemicals in the human environment. The 1974 edition has an excellent introduction.

A Guide to Alternative Medicine by Robert Eagle (1980). Published in conjunction with the BBC Radio 4 series, *Alternative Medicine*. A well written guide to the principal areas of practice.

Chemical Victims by Richard Mackarness (1980). A good British introduction to clinical ecology. Informative on problems with food and those chemical cleansers. Recommended.

Allergies — Your Hidden Enemy by Theron G. Randolph and Ralph W. Moss (1981). Case studies and information on the general field of Clinical Ecology, with practical advice, written in American.

Medicines — A Guide for Everybody by Peter Parish (1976). Every household should have a ready source of information on drugs. This one is informative and usable.

Martindale: The Extra Pharmacopaeia ed. by J. Reynolds (1982). This is *the* source reference work on drugs. It is comprehensive, detailed, and very expensive. Your local library should have a copy if you want to investigate any pharmaceutical product.

Cured to Death — the Effects of Prescription Drugs by Arabella Melville and Colin Johnson (1982). We would like everyone who believes that medicine has 'the answer', or that health is available over the chemist's counter to read our book. It has nothing in it specifically about hay fever.

The Limits To Growth (1972). The report of the Club of Rome's project on the predicament of mankind. The investigations carried out, the methods used, and the inescapable conclusions. All in an easy to understand form with the minimum of technicality. This book should be more widely read than the Bible if humanity is to have any future.

The Patient, not the Cure: The Challenge of Homoeopathy (1976). Marjorie Blackie was physician to the Queen and the book contains a useful discussion of hay fever and its treatment.

References

Allen, F. *et al.*, Grass pollen concentrations in the UK. *J. Roy. Soc. Hlth.*, *103*, 1983, 85–7.

Bagni, N. *et al.*, City spore concentrations in the European Economic Community. *Clinical Allergy*, 1976, *6*, 61–69.

Blackley, C.H. *Hayfever: its causes, treatment, and effective prevention*. London: Balliere, 1880.

Breeds, J.A. Effects of hay fever on students' work and examination performance. *Commun. Med.*, June 1972, 255.

Cuthbert, O.D., *Clinical Allergy, 11*, 1981.

Davies, R.R. and Smith, L.P. Weather and the grass pollen content of the air. *Clin. All*, 1973, *3*, 95–108.

Eaton, K. *et al.*, *Allergy Therapeutics*. London: Balliere Tindall, 1982.

Freedman, S.O. in *Clinical Immunology*. New York: Harper & Row, 1971.

Harland, R.W. The management of hay fever in general practice. *J. Roy. Coll. Gen. Pract.*, *29*, 1979, 265–286.

Hyde, H.A. Atmospheric pollen grains and spores in relation to allergy. *Clinical Allergy, 3*, 1973, 109–126.

Jones, R.L. and Jenkins, M.D. Plant responses to homoeopathic remedies. *Brit. Hom. J., 70*, 1981, 120–135.

Kennedy, C.O. Do homoeopathic remedies work in practice? *Brit. Hom. J., 69*, 1980, 6–11.

Knox, R.B. *Pollen and Allergy*. Edward Arnold.

Lau, B.H., *et al.*, Effect of acupuncture on allergic rhinitis. *Am. J. Chin. Med., 3*, 1975, 263–70.

Martindale: The Extra Pharmacopaeia. 28th Ed., 1983.

Middleton, E. *et al., Eds., Allergy: Principles and Practice. (2nd. Ed.)* St. Louis: Mosby, 1983.

Miller, A.C.M.L. A trial of hyposensitization in 1974/5 in the treatment of hay fever using glutaraldehyde-pollen tyrosine adsorbate. *Clin. All.* 1976, *6*, 557–561.

Milner & Tees, *Clinical Allergy, 2*, 1972, 83.

Moyle, A. *Nature Cure for Asthma and Hay Fever*. Wellingborough: Thorsons, 1975.

Puhakka, H., & Rantanen, T. Cryotherapy as a method of treatment in allergic and vasomotor rhinitis. *J. Laryng. & Otol., 91*, 1977, 535.

Rands, D.A. and Godfrey, R.C. Side effects of desensitization for allergy — a general practice survey. *J. Roy. Coll. Gen. Pract.*, 1983, *33*, 647–649.

Skegg, D, *et al.*, Antihistamines and motorcycle accidents. *Brit. Med. J., i*, 1979, 917.

Watts, G. Years before the mast. *World Med.*, June 1979, 35–41.

Royal College of General Practitioners: Morbidity Statistics from General Practice, 1955
ditto, 1970.

Non-sedative antihistamines: terfenadine and astemizole. *Drug and Therapeutics Bulletin*, 1984, *22*, No. 6.

Appendix I

Principal Sources* of Allergy at Various Locations

Place	*Allergens* (in order of importance)
London	Grass Pollens
	Plane/Silver birch tree pollen
	Alternaria (a mould growing on cereal crops)
Derby	Grass pollens
	Cladosporium (a mould on rotting vegetation)
	Sporobolomyces (a fungus on leaf surfaces)
Orkney	Hay dust
	Horse, sheep, cat
	Fungi
Finland	Birch pollen
	Grass pollen
	Mugwort
Nepal	Mixed threshings
	Pollens
Kuwait	*Proposis spicigera* (an introduced tree)
	Chenopod (a native bush)
	Moulds
NE USA	Ragwort (a weed on cultivated land)
	Grass pollens

*Note House dust mite allergy has been excluded from this table. It is one of the principal causes of allergy everywhere, all the year round.

Appendix II

Principal Allergenic Grasses

Common Name	Latin Name	Pollen season	Location
Timothy Grass	Phleum pratense	June-August	Meadows, hayfield
Cocksfoot	Dactylis glomerata	June-September	Meadows
Rye Grass	Lolium perenne	May-August	Lawns, pasture
Meadow Fescue	Festuca pratensis	June—August	Meadows
Yorkshire Fog	Holcus lanatus	May-August	General
Scented Vernal	Anthoxanthum odoratum	April-June	Generally abundant

Different species of grass are abundant in different parts of the country, and the probable culprits in grass pollen allergy will be found near the victim's home or work-place. Many allergens are shared by different species of grasses, so anyone who reacts to one grass is likely to react to others.

Appendix III

Average daily grass pollen counts, London, 1961-70

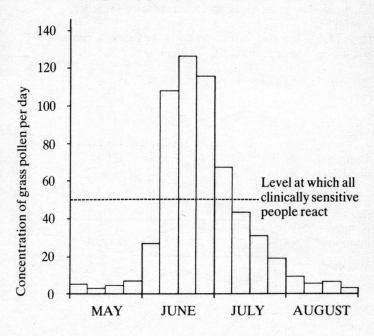

Mean pollen levels (grains/m^3) per day weeks (approx.)

Month	1	2	3	4
May	5·0	3·0	4·5	6·5
June	26·5	108·0	126·6	116·0
July	67·7	43·4	31·4	19·4
August	9·4	5·9	6·8	3·5

Figures calculated from data in table 1 of Davies, R.R. & Smith, L.P.: Weather and the grass pollen content of the air, *Clinical Allergy*, 1973, *3*, 95-108.

Appendix IV

Fluctuations in grass pollen levels in relation to weather
conditions
(From J. Mullins *et al*, "Grass pollen in the Bristol Channel
Region", *Clinical Allergy*, 1977, 7, p.394.)

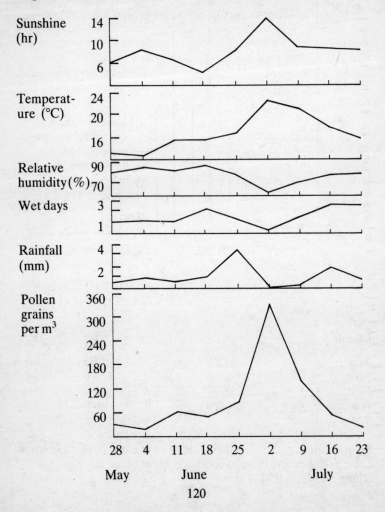

Appendix V

Seasons of Principal Plant Allergens (Southern England)

Month	Source	Duration
January	household moulds	all year round
February	hazel	mid-April
" (late)	elm	late April
March	"	"
April	ash	entire month
"	birch	mid-May
" (late)	plane	late May
May	grasses	August
June	nettles	August
July	moulds*	October

Thereafter, no new sources.

*mainly growing on cereal crops

Appendix VI

Annual Variations

Annual pollen levels 1975-79 Cardiff
Showing annual variation of 12:1 (Birch).
Data from Dr John Mullins, Asthma Research Unit,
Sully Hospital, South Glamorgan.

Appendix VII

Common Recognised Industrial Allergens

Cotton and flax dust
Isocyanates in polyurethane foam insulation, adhesives, etc
Laboratory animals and insects
Colophony in soldering fluxes and hot melt glues
Enzymes in biological detergents*
complex salts of platinum in platinum refiners
Flour and grains in bakers, millers, farmers, etc
Epoxy resin curing agents in adhesives and coatings
Wood dusts in carpenters etc
Metals such as cobalt and nickel used in plating and steels
Drugs in drug manufacture, e.g. antibiotics
Micro-organisms from contaminated humidifiers
Formaldehyde in adhesives and moulding mixtures

*In Norway, all domestic washing products containing enzymes carry warnings about health hazards, particularly allergenicity. In Britain, almost all generally available automatic washing powders contain enzymes and are liable to produce allergic reactions, despite the absence of warnings.

Appendix VIII

Avoidance of Exposure to House Dust Mite
(Advice provided by the Glasgow Homoeopathic Hospital)

BEDS AND BEDDING.

The most important consideration.

Mattresses should be of solid foam, covered with a plastic or PVC cover. This cover prevents any penetrance of the mite into the foam, and has the advantage that it is easily wiped clean. Pillows may be washable, non-allergic or solid foam.

Acrylan or polyester underblankets are available which counteract the cold feel of the plastic cover and prevent slipping of the overlying bedclothes.

All sheets, blankets, quilts or downies must be readily washable and should be thoroughly washed and aired every two to three months. Materials such as polyester/cotton, acrylan and dacron are ideal. Using these materials it is possible to wash the underblanket, blankets and downies in the morning, and even in winter-time, have them dried and back on the bed by evening. This saves having to duplicate blankets, quilts etc in order to achieve the mandatory two-three monthly wash.

The base of the bed should be of simple springs or wooden slats. No upholstered divan bases.

OTHER POINTS TO WATCH.

Soft toys such as teddy bears and golliwogs can become infested with house dust mites as readily as bedding. These should therefore be made of washable materials and treated similarly to the bed.

Sufferers from house dust mite allergy should not sleep in or sit or bounce on other beds unless these have been treated in a similar fashion to their own.

If there is more than one bed in the patient's bedroom, then these other beds must be treated also otherwise there will be an aerosol effect of house dust mites from these beds with every movement of their occupants.

Children must be advised not to bounce on upholstered furniture, crawl under beds or hide in wardrobes.

Vacuuming of carpets must not be done in the presence of the house dust sufferer, and preferably not within two hours of him being around.

If the sufferer is the housewife, it is advisable that all the beds in the house be treated so that she does not become exposed when dealing with the beds of other members of the family. She should also either get someone else to do the vacuuming for her, or else wear an efficient mask while performing this task.

Ducted-air central heating must be avoided as this spreads house dust mites througout the whole atmosphere of the house.

HOLIDAYS

The problem of sleeping arrangements while on holiday are easily dealt with. The patient should take with him his own pillow, a large sheet of good quality plastic, and a washable sleeping bag (and blankets if desired). The plastic is spread over the entire bed on which he will sleep, and the sleeping bag and pillow placed on top. Ideally there should be no one else sharing his room.

THE 3D SLIMMING DIET
by Dr. Michael Spira

At last! Lose weight permanently and reduce the risk of heart disease and cancer with this new medically approved diet.

Approved by world health experts, THE 3D DIET is suitable for all the family, and easy to follow anywhere, not just at home.

THE 3 DO'S
You do lose weight safely and permanently.
You do something positive for your health (i.e. you reduce your risk of disease, especially coronary heart disease and some cancers).
You do eat nutritionally sound and balanced meals which are delicious and varied.

THE 3 DON'TS
You don't eat too many calories.
You don't eat too many saturated fats.
You don't eat too much cholesterol.

Here are carefully analysed facts about food and low cholesterol meals.

A life plan towards maintaining weight loss and creating a new life style.

0 552 12366 8   £1.75

THE BEVERLY HILLS EXERCISE BOOK
by Roberta Krech with Bill Libby

YOU CAN LEARN THE SECRETS OF BEAUTY AND FITNESS THAT, UNTIL NOW, ONLY THE ELITE COULD AFFORD.

From her exclusive Beverly Hills salon, physical fitness and skin-care expert Roberta Krech invites you to experience the simple, natural exercise programme that gives her rich and famous clients their youthful looks and slim, supple figures.

Ms Krech will show you how to 'steal' a few minutes here and there throughout your day for the quick and easy exercises that will keep you trim, toned and energized. Wherever you are, from morning till midnight, her fabulous star-proven system will shape up your entire body — face and neck, shoulders and upper arms, bust and back, waist and abdomen, hips and buttocks, thighs and calves, ankles and feet . . . and there's never a boring callisthenic to do!

With personal beauty tips and professional skin care instructions, plus exercises to share and relaxation techniques, THE BEVERLY HILLS EXERCISE BOOK allows you to attain the radiant and glowing beauty of the fashionable women of Beverly Hills.

0 552 12158 4

£1.75

ARTHRITIS
Relief Beyond Drugs
by Rachel Carr

If you are one of the many thousands of people who suffer from arthritis you will know that drug therapy is essential for certain conditions – but by itself that is not always enough. Impaired mobility and the emotional effects of chronic pain can be greatly reduced, and sufferers helped to come to terms with their condition by following a daily routine of the stretching and limbering, deep breathing and relaxation exercises described in this book.

Rachel Carr, at one time severely disabled by osteo-arthritis, now tells you what simple techniques she used herself. The exercises are straightforward and varied so that every arthritis sufferer can benefit from them.

0 552 99033 7   £1.95

THE POCKET HOLIDAY DOCTOR
by Caroline Chapman and Caroline Lucas BM BcH

All the do's and don'ts for a healthy holiday . . .

How to keep the family free from holiday hazards . . .

How to cope with sickness, diarrhoea, sunburn, bites, fever, etc . . .

Zero hour – when to recognise that you *must* have a doctor, and how to find one in any language . . .

One of the authors of THE POCKET HOLIDAY DOCTOR, Caroline Chapman, found herself in a mother's nightmare. In an idyllic holiday home, her ten-year-old child developed a temperature of 103° and had diarrhoea so severe that she was passing blood. They had no transport. The nearest telephone was half a mile away, the nearest doctor ten miles and he couldn't speak English.

There and then Caroline Chapman vowed that if her daughter pulled through, she would write a book offering practical advice.

Here, from Caroline Chapman and Dr Caroline Lucas, is a book for emergencies of all kinds, from the sting of a jelly fish, to a possible outbreak of cholera.

0 552 12195 9   £1.25

A SELECTION OF HEALTH, DIET AND PHYSICAL FITNESS TITLES AVAILABLE FROM CORGI BOOKS

While every effort is made to keep prices low, it is sometimes necessary to increase prices at short notice. Corgi Books reserve the right to show new retail prices on covers which may differ from those previously advertised in the text or elsewhere.

The prices shown below were correct at the time of going to press.

☐ 11033 7	THE SUPER ENERGY DIET	Dr Robert Atkins with Shirley Motter Linde	£1.25
☐ 99033 7	ARTHRITIS	Rachel Carr	£1.95
☐ 10336 5	THE MAGIC OF HONEY	Barbara Cartland	£1.50
☐ 12195 9	THE POCKET HOLIDAY DOCTOR	Caroline Chapman and Dr Caroline Lucas	£1.25
☐ 99070 1	WORK THAT BODY!	Jackie Genova	£2.95
☐ 99044 2	THE HERPES BOOK	Richard Hamilton M.D.	£2.95
☐ 12379 X	JUDITH HANN'S TOTAL HEALTH PLAN	Judith Hann	£1.75
☑ 12554 7	THE PETER PAN SYNDROME	Dr Dan Kiley	£1.95
☐ 12158 4	THE BEVERLY HILLS EXERCISE BOOK	Roberta Krech	£1.75
☐ 99011 6	SEXUAL HEALTH AND FITNESS FOR WOMEN	Kathryn Lance and Maria Agardy	£1.95
☐ 11954 7	HOMEOPATHIC MEDICINE AT HOME	Maesimund B. Panos M.D. and Jane Heinlich	£2.95
☐ 12220 3	GROWING PAINS	Claire Rayner	£4.95
☐ 12366 8	THE 3-D SLIMMING DIET	Michael Spira	£1.75
☐ 12377 3	THE COMPLETE SCARSDALE MEDICAL DIET	Herman Tarnower and Samm Sinclair Baker	£1.95
☐ 98058 7	YOGA AND NUTRITION	Kareen Zebroff	£1.25
☐ 98059 5	BEAUTY THROUGH YOGA	Kareen Zebroff	£1.25

ORDER FORM

All these books are available at your book shop or newsagent, or can be ordered direct from the publisher. Just tick the titles you want and fill in the form below.

CORGI BOOKS, Cash Sales Department, P.O. Box 11, Falmouth, Cornwall.

Please send cheque or postal order, no currency.

Please allow cost of book(s) plus the following for postage and packing:

U.K. Customers — Allow 55p for the first book, 22p for the second book and 14p for each additional book ordered, to a maximum charge of £1.75.

B.F.P.O. and Eire — Allow 55p for the first book, 22p for the second book plus 14p per copy for the next seven books, thereafter 8p per book.

Overseas Customers — Allow £1.00 for the first book and 25p per copy for each additional book.

NAME (Block Letters) ....

ADDRESS ....

....